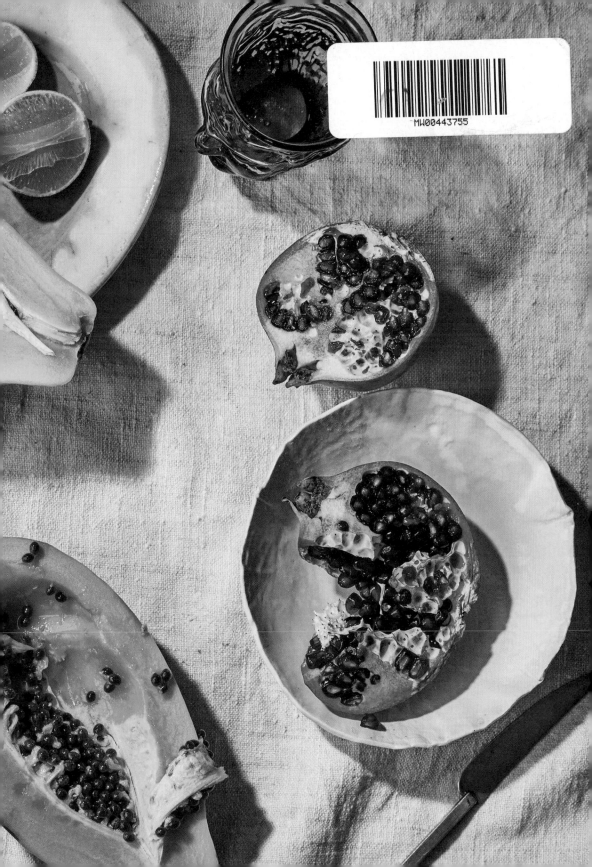

Ayurvedic Rituals

Wisdom, Recipes + the Ancient Art of Self-Care

For the seekers

Chasca Summerville

Hardie Grant

BOOKS

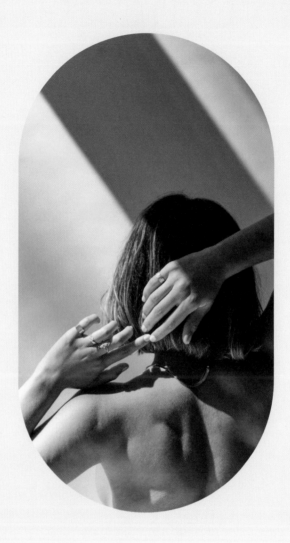

This book uses metric cup measurements, i.e. 250 ml (8½ fl oz) for 1 cup; in the US a cup is 8 fl oz, just smaller, and American cooks should be generous in their cup measurements; in the UK a cup is 10 fl oz and British cooks should be scant with their cup measurements.

It also uses a 20 ml (¾ fl oz) tablespoon; cooks using a 15 ml (½ fl oz) tablespoon should be generous with their tablespoon measurements.

Contents

An invitation to explore

I invite you to come on a journey to explore ancient, altruistic and intrinsically primal philosophies that inspire a sensual way of living – a lifestyle infused with ritual and poetry, where life becomes an expression of creativity and colour, imbued with our connection to Mother Nature and all of her inhabitants. This journey together allows us to develop an intuitive relationship with the plant kingdom and the natural world; to honour ourselves and all living beings with love and compassion; to craft a lifestyle that nourishes the multi-dimensional aspects of who you are; and to create an existence on planet earth that does not destruct her wild nature. This is Ayurveda – the Art of Living.

Ayurveda provides the channel for you to connect with your body, mind and spirit on a path of empowerment where you can intuitively recognise and harmonise daily imbalances, ultimately unlocking an invaluable sense of freedom, health and vitality. This is a journey in becoming your own healer. There is no greater state of being than to live in the home of a body that is balanced, a mind that is content and a soul that is satisfied. It is my driving force to share this ancient wisdom to liberate you and impart the tools you need to access this form of bliss.

For me, Ayurveda has been a journey of deep self-discovery that has allowed me to understand myself beyond my wildest dreams. I have learnt not only to accept, but to embrace as blessings, the more challenging aspects of myself and my experiences through life. Throughout this process, I have been able to

discover all of the wisdom I have gained as a result of my experiences, which ultimately course through my veins and make me the person I am today. Ayurveda uncovers the delicate nature of balance and how every negative has a positive, or every weakness a strength. This understanding frees the shackles of unresolved trauma, allowing us to open our hearts to unconditional gratitude. There is no greater way to slow down and connect with the soul than by returning to our ancient roots and adopting practices that allow us to become fully aware and utterly present.

Ayurveda is centred around living sustainably, minimising our carbon footprint, reducing our waste and living within our means. Right now the planet needs our help. Research and science have stated that it is not unreasonable to think that humans are facing extinction, based on our modern lifestyle and the rate at which we consume finite natural resources, not to mention the rapid decline of our fellow species and nature itself. By implementing the practices within this book, you can drastically reduce your impact on the planet and access a zero-waste lifestyle. Our current way of living and the rate at which we consume is no longer an option for us; each of us has a responsibility to turn this around, as a necessity – and with the right resources, I can assure you the changes are widely accessible and vastly rewarding.

With so many compelling philosophies available on how to live your life and the constructs by which to live it, pay attention to those that sing out to you, that spark something deep within that makes you want to explore a little further, that make all of the pieces of your soul click together – that moment where everything just makes sense. The greatest lessons will send you back to your self and provoke a passion within that fuels your desire and thirst for knowledge. When you have this, then you know you are on the right path. The deeper my exploration of Ayurveda has taken me over the years, the more closely I appreciate the interconnectedness of all the aspects of this truly holistic, vast and expansive body of knowledge by which I am truly grateful to live by.

Alchemy is transformation in its truest essence. Whether this is the transformation of a plant into medicine, food into energy or a negative experience into a positive one – we all have the ability to transform, evolve and reshape our patterns and our way of thinking. I urge you to fall in love with yourself and all of the cracks and crevices of life. Trust in knowing that everything is perfect. Regardless of how you see yourself, know that your body is beautiful, that it is the most incredible and amazing thing you will ever own, there is no other like it, you are one of a kind and you have so much to be grateful for. Never forget how wildly capable you are.

This book is my homage to Ayurveda – a timeless science that has taught me how to live consciously, liberate myself from suffering and access ultimate health and wellbeing while living symbiotically with nature. The teachings in this book are not my own; they stem from a five-thousand-year-old body of knowledge passed down from the sages of India that explores the rich tapestry of herbalism, meditation, mindfulness, yoga, plant-based cooking, gut health, digestion, self-care rituals, living within nature, honouring the planet, and beyond.

My intention is to utilise the knowledge of Ayurveda to help you create rituals that will allow you to:

o   Live sustainably.

o   Flood your body with nutrition.

o   Gain a state of health that inspires boundless energy, deep sleep and a positive outlook.

o   Access the plant kingdom to craft your own personal care products as a means of bypassing anything toxic.

o   Adopt self-care practices that allow you to slow down and connect with your body.

o   Find solace in daily rituals that honour both your physical and mental wellbeing.

o   Unlock the tools to prevent disease and eliminate the need to cure it.

o   Live in tune with nature and the seasons.

o   Understand and utilise plants respectfully.

o   Read and heal imbalances on a daily basis.

o   Listen and communicate with your body and mind in a way that only you can.

And by doing so – ultimately access your highest potential for health and happiness.

May your journey into the vast waters of Ayurveda be filled with knowledge, wisdom, exploration, playfulness, joy and liberation.

THE SCIENCE
OF LIFE

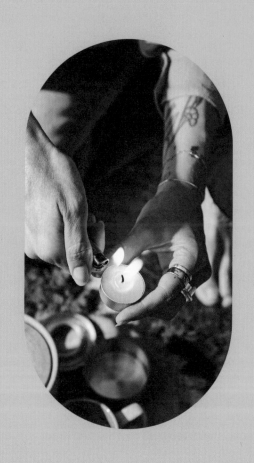

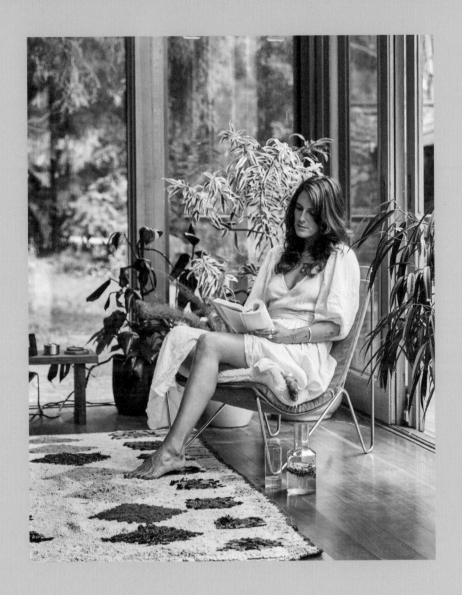

Introducing Ayurveda

Ayurveda is known as the 'Mother of All Healing' and has deep roots in ancient Vedic wisdom. Thousands of years before modern medicine was designed to solve problems created by poor health and disease, the sages of India discovered Ayurveda – a sophisticated science that understands the relationship between the body + mind, as well as our place within nature and how to access plants, energy, ritual, the seasons and our environment to cultivate health and wellbeing on both a physical and spiritual level. Ayurveda is a system of healing that considers physical constitution, emotional nature and spiritual outlook as a complete package.

Translated as the 'Science of Life' (ayur = life; veda = science), Ayurveda is the original system of holistic healthcare, providing insight on diet, lifestyle, herbal medicine, meditation, yoga, living in alignment with nature and the seasons, and methods for both preventing and healing disease. Ayurveda paved the way for alternative modalities we know and love today such as Chinese medicine, acupuncture, naturopathy, homeopathy and herbalism.

Born out of a culture that is rich in spiritual wisdom and tradition, Ayurveda was taught through poetry and song long before it was first documented thousands of years BC in the oldest known language, 'Sanskrit'. Literature written in Sanskrit, which is known as the 'perfect language', has a deep intent behind it, with every letter and word designed to resonate a potent vibration. Meditation was also used to access and share the philosophies of Ayurveda

and it was through these practices that India became known as the epicentre of spirituality, magnetising anyone seeking peace, health and vitality. It's no surprise that Western icons such as The Beatles, Beat poets like Allen Ginsberg, and the whole Sannyasin movement sought refuge in the land of peace and tranquillity.

Ayurveda is a holistic science that addresses all aspects of life, including the body, mind and emotions. It respects each person's unique needs and tailors treatments to complement their strengths and weaknesses. Ayurveda values medicine and diet as complementary rather than separate, unlike modern medicine, which generally aims to treat symptoms rather than causes and often neglects the importance of diet and mental health. Prevention is key in Ayurveda, with an entire diet and lifestyle system based upon creating an internal environment that supports powerful digestion, nourishment of all tissues, strong immunity, vitality and longevity. If this perfect harmony is disrupted, Ayurveda provides us with the tools to recognise symptoms intuitively at a very early stage so that we can adjust our diet and lifestyle to restore balance.

> ## 'When diet is wrong, medicine is of no use. When diet is correct, medicine is of no need.'
>
> — AYURVEDIC PROVERB
> from Charaka Samhita

Also known as the 'Art of Living', Ayurveda has many beautiful rituals we can adopt in our daily lives that work to restore balance and nourish the body, mind and soul on a deep level. These practices honour nature, inspire us to slow down, connect with ourselves and reduce the detrimental effects of living a fast-paced life while allowing us to tune in and live in sync with ancient traditions designed to serve humankind and the planet.

In addition to the health benefits of Ayurveda, philosophies of non-violence towards all beings, animals and the planet are at the root of the lifestyle practices, meaning that we have the tools to minimise our footprint on the earth – reducing the devastating effects of environmental destruction in an age when this has never been more necessary.

Through living in alignment with your environment, you will develop an appreciation and understanding of nature like never before. Nature provides the foundations for life. Plant foods flourish at a time when they are needed by the body to complement the changes in weather. Seasons work together to provide balance and allow space for the intrinsic patterns of life to exist. Nature provides all of the nourishment we need to thrive, through herbs, spices, grains, seeds, legumes, fruit and vegetables. It is up to us to work harmoniously with her to complement what is naturally abundant. It is this flow, this dance, that allows us to live a balanced, effortless life, in tune with the natural rhythms of our environment.

As a holistic lifestyle, Ayurveda provides a foundation from which we can live our lives with effortless grace. By honouring Ayurvedic philosophies, you have the ability to access:

o   A diet crafted to your individual, ever-changing needs that flows throughout the seasons to complement what is naturally abundant.

o   A lifestyle imbued with ancient rituals for self-care that nurture and nourish the body, mind and spirit, giving access to a greater sense of worth, love and respect for ourselves.

o   A spiritual anchor that supports your mental health and emotional wellbeing through practices that allow you to live a mindful existence, armed with the strength to overcome stress and trauma while exploring the beauty of the bounty that surrounds us.

o   A relationship with nature that allows us to live in harmony with our habitat while minimising our footprint on the planet.

o   A radiant state of health that shines from the inside out through practices that strengthen immunity, foster longevity, promote vitality and inspire energy.

o   An appreciation and love for life like never before.

The place of Ayurveda in the modern world

How does a system of healing that was developed many thousands of years ago still have resonance in an age where nothing is as it was? If you look at the fundamentals of Ayurveda, you will find that the philosophies are timeless - in order to embody true health, we must possess a calm mind, be in control of our emotions, consume a nutrient-rich diet, live a life of fulfillment and service, in attunement with the natural world that surrounds us, while nourishing our body, mind and spirit through self-care practices and movement.

This style of living allows us to deep dive into the pool of health and wellness while forming a sensual bond with ourselves and our environment regardless of our age or sex, where we live or in which century we exist. Over the last five thousand years, there has not been one day where Ayurveda has not been relevant, nor have any of the philosophies of Ayurveda been brought undone. In fact, as modern science progresses, studies are being brought to light daily that provide scientific backing for the incredible benefits of the Ayurvedic lifestyle in every realm, from meditation to herbal medication.

In the modern world we have been birthed into a culture of 'go, go, go'. The romance once found in the pleasures of the 'simple life' has gone – slow days were lived in alignment with the sun, a bounty of foods full of life force were harvested straight from the garden and fresh meals were prepared from scratch. We took the time to nourish our bodies with practices like daily oil massage and quietened the mind with long meditation sessions; we used our bodies as our mode of transport and were active throughout the day. This naturalistic way of living has been flipped completely upside down as the standard expectation to fulfil fulltime work often requires us to rush off early in cars, sit all day long staring at digital screens – with artificial light wreaking havoc on our hormonal systems – and unconsciously cram highly processed fast food into our mouths as we work around the clock to meet what is required of us. In this state of high-intensity living, we can easily neglect our need for nutrition, replacing it with quick and easy modern products that make lots of promises but sadly rarely deliver.

As we ingest and consume toxic ingredients (through both our mouth and skin), our bodies enter a state of inflammation (or Pitta aggravation, see page 24) that creates a breeding ground for disease to manifest. We are then introduced to a cycle of synthetic medications to reduce the inflammation that then install their own set of side-effects and by-products which then require further help to resolve, and the cycle revolves continually, with no light at the end of the tunnel. The key to freeing yourself from this self-perpetuating cycle of disease is to work to remove the root cause of suffering, and this can be done in the modern world through the use of Ayurveda. By implementing some practices that help to reduce stress and equip you with the tools to protect yourself from emotional turmoil, by adopting some healthier diet practices and improving your self-care routines, you can harness the power of ultimate health and liberation from disease.

The value of this ancient lifestyle has a greater poignancy than ever before, as, across the planet, we are faced with more and more alarming health crises and mental health disorders due to the nature of our rapid evolution. As life speeds up, it's crucial to slow down. It is this form of balance that keeps us grounded. When we are moving too fast, we must slow; when we are burdened with fear, we must fly; when we have too much heat, we must cool; when we are shackled with lack of motivation, we must act; when we are burnt out, we must rest. It's this exchange between polarities that keeps us balanced while also stretching the limits of our comfort zone to make space for spiritual growth and to enable a lust for life to flourish.

Through adopting Ayurvedic principles in your life, you will gain the intuition to recognise all kinds of imbalances on a daily basis and pinpoint where they came from, why they're showing up and how you can rectify them through your diet, lifestyle, ritual and self-care practices. Tapping into this form of intuition creates a poetic and romantic relationship between your body, mind and soul that allows you to fully understand yourself and utilise the knowledge of what does and doesn't work for you.

As we continue to burn out, our hearts and minds are opening to ancient practices.

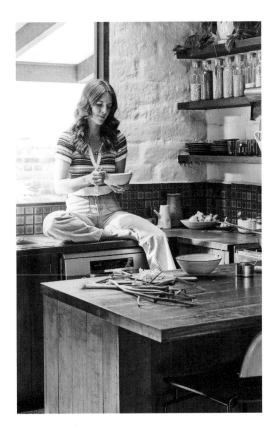

Becoming your own healer

If you find yourself feeling overwhelmed by the endless barrage of diet trends that come and go, each with conflicting messages on health, trust in knowing that Ayurveda provides a health solution that has stood the test of time – thousands of years in fact – with diet principles that have not faltered since their inception.

Ayurveda embraces nourishing, balanced, wholesome foods that come from the earth and flood your body with warmth and nutrition, keeping your digestive fire alive, providing energy and vitality, and working both to prevent and heal disease on a daily basis. Once you know your constitution (Dosha), you can begin to work with the foods recommended in this book to look and feel your best. No more calorie counting, food-journalling, meal replacements, diet shakes or frozen meals! Just truly delicious, well-balanced, heart-warming bowls of nourishment

ADAPTING AYURVEDA TO SUIT YOUR NEEDS AND LIFESTYLE

We are all unique beings who have our own special blueprint, with certain energies, imbalances, DNA, upbringings, spiritual and karmic responsibilities, injuries, emotional and physical trauma, and so much more. There is no possible way to design a single system for restoring balance within every person when we all embody such unique differences, which can fluctuate daily.

We must look at the individual, respect their constitution, identify their symptoms and the

energy or Dosha with which they are associated, then utilise the qualities of the counter-balancing Dosha to restore harmony. It's that simple, and everyone can use it, everywhere, every day. When you begin to understand this philosophy, you will be able to work with your body and have much more success than even a qualified practitioner could achieve for you, as only you can have such a deep understanding of yourself. Recognise that pain and symptoms are the gateway, the portal from the interior that resides beneath the surface, shining a spotlight to enable our internal compass to navigate our experience of health.

Does it feel like you have tried every skincare regime on the market and you just can't seem to get it right? Or perhaps you're simply looking for that extra glow that doesn't require makeup or synthetic chemicals. Ayurveda can help you discover the individual needs of your skin type and how to bring balance to any problem areas through a bounty of beautiful rituals that balance inflammation, restore lustre and even prevent the signs of ageing, all through natural, edible products that you can make yourself. Ayurveda believes that if it's not good enough to eat, it shouldn't go on your skin!

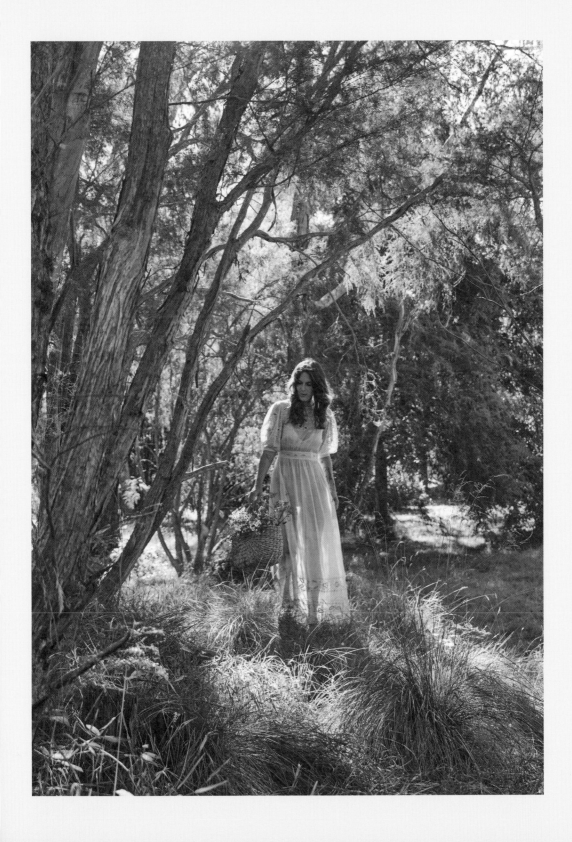

It's all about syncing up and diving into what's going on beneath the surface of your body. When we spend our lives rushing from one place to another, distracting ourselves by having multiple things on the go at all times, it's hard to create space to tap into the messages our body is trying to send us. We neglect this deep form of connection with ourselves and instead look for quick fixes to silence the symptoms that show what is really going on inside.

In the modern world, if we have an outbreak on our skin, our first response is to rush into a chemist and look for some kind of cream to get rid of this eyesore. What we should be doing is questioning what has caused the outbreak – was it a new food?, a place we ate?, or perhaps a skincare product that our body is rejecting? The message we're being sent is our body's way of telling us that something we have ingested is toxic and needs to be avoided. We hold such an incredible potential for intuition but fail to harness this innate power. All of the health concerns you have ever experienced are opportunities from which you can learn, messages from within that help to guide you so that you are only eating and living in a way that complements your best opportunity for true health and wellbeing. Imagine if instead of being upset, angry or irritated when you experienced a health burden, you instead expressed gratitude for the message and looked deep within to uncover the root cause so that you could avoid it entirely in the future. This is the ultimate tool for self-actualisation and the key to boundless health and vitality.

Understanding the paradigm between our innate constitution (Dosha) and our imbalances allows us to become fluent in the language of our body.

You can open up the channels of communication between your body and mind through patience, respect and connection to self. So many of the elements of the modern world distract us from our intuitive abilities. We possess the potential to decipher exactly what foods we are in need of, the subtle changes in the environment that play an important role in our lifestyle practices, right through to the parts of our bodies which may be suffering and in need of attention. When we strip away the layers of social conditioning, and the practices that result, we are able to return to our true state of being.

Did you know?

For someone experiencing extreme heat in the body, which may look like fever, inflammation, skin irritations (acne, rosacea or dermatitis), diarrhoea, reflux etc., it makes sense that the priority should be on cooling down the system with things like alkaline meals, bitter greens, aloe vera juice and calming teas like mint, fennel and chamomile while avoiding heating/stimulating substances like chilli, caffeine, alcohol, fried foods etc.

For someone experiencing extreme lethargy, chronic fatigue, sluggish digestion, chills etc., a bit of spice might be just the ticket to kickstart their system by generating some internal heat to get things moving.

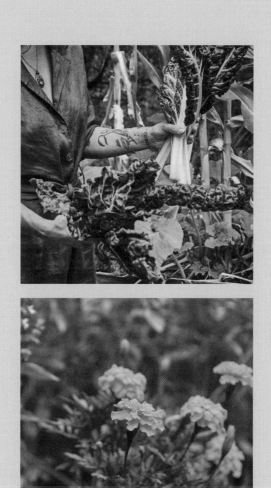

I personally suffered from debilitating period pain from the age of fifteen and felt that I had tried everything I could to get a handle on it. I was booked in for intrusive surgery that came with its own risks and could possibly leave scar tissue that has the potential to manifest into a plethora of other health concerns later down the line. With the wisdom of **Ayurveda**, I was able to direct my energy inward and ask the question my body had been aching to answer for over a decade. Through this process, I discovered that I had been neglecting the very core of my **womanhood** residing in the womb – through poor choices in sexual partners, self-sabotage, several hormonally interfering drugs, unresolved issues relating to the lineage of women that had been before me, neglect of the seasons of the menstrual cycle and not allowing myself time to rest and recuperate during menses. All of these responses came flooding to me once I sat and simply **asked the question**.

I began to implement all of the knowledge I had gained and I was astounded by the **transformation**. I could not believe the profound changes that began to **blossom within**. I had resolved the pain within four months and cancelled my surgery. After years of trying everything under the sun, all I had to do was sit, **connect with my body**, ask what it needed, and act on it. In having this realisation, and finding myself liberated from the debilitating pain, I was able to express deep gratitude for the pain that had burdened me for most of my adult life. I now understand that pain is merely a message for our consideration and that when it arises, there is **healing** to be done.

Beginning your journey with Ayurveda

Adopting an Ayurvedic lifestyle may seem a little intimidating at first but as you begin to understand the fundamentals and deepen your practice, you will find a rhythm that complements your schedule and allows you to get the most out of each and every day.

Simply by beginning to apply some of the philosophies that resonate with you and your mental, spiritual and physical health goals, you will begin to notice a difference in your wellbeing that you can then continue to build on over time. Ayurveda supports daily ritual, discipline and consistency. You may need to be a little more organised at first and plan ahead but over time this will become second nature. Design a guideline that works for you and try to practise it as regularly as possible. The more time you invest, the more effortlessly you will find yourself gravitating towards the practices as the benefits begin to blossom and bloom within. It's the practices we choose today that inspire how we feel tomorrow.

Clean eating, self-care, meditation and movement will all ensure deep, restful and restorative sleep that will impart more energy for the daily practices, which you can introduce in small increments and build on over time. As your energy clears, you will feel more drawn to longer meditation practices as you seek more of the internal peace that comes from having this spiritual anchor. As you find your rhythm in the kitchen, you'll crave the buzz that comes from eating wholesome nutrient-dense meals made with love. As your skin, eyes, hair and nails begin to glow, you will respect products that are completely natural and infused with the healing powers of the plant kingdom and nothing but! Once you find your groove, you can expect to gain abundant energy, deep, restful sleep, vibrant eyes, luscious hair, glowing skin, a healthy body, strong immunity – and, best of all, a happy, content and satisfied mind.

See if you can approach your relationship with Ayurveda as an adventure, indulge in the moments of bliss you experience, and savour them – and keep coming back to your sources of inspiration – wanting to cultivate a life of physical, emotional and spiritual wellbeing.

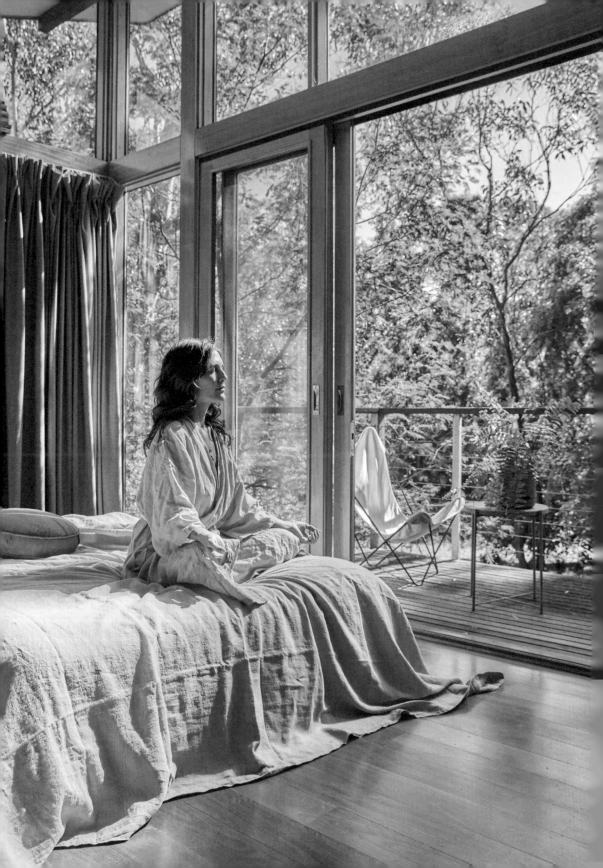

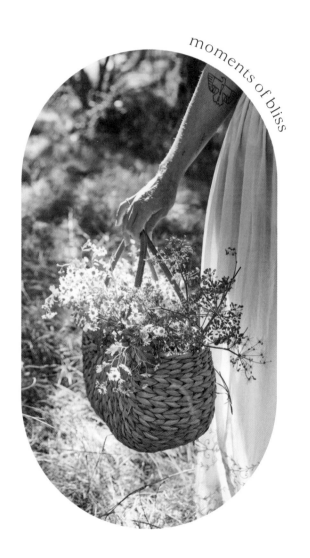

moments of bliss

THE DOSHAS

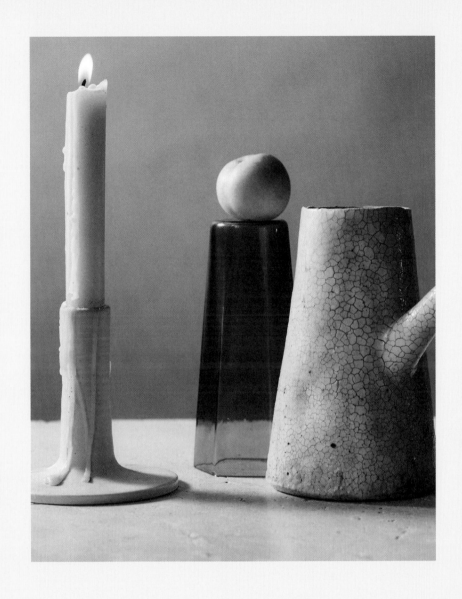

2

Vata, Pitta + Kapha

The secret to understanding Ayurveda is through learning the subtle energies and qualities of the Doshas. Ayurveda recognises three basic types of energy, known as the Three Doshas (Vata, Pitta and Kapha), which are present in everyone and everything.

Each of the three Doshas has its own identity based on a combination of the Five Great Elements (Space, Air, Fire, Water + Earth). Each of these elements possesses certain qualities that give the Doshas their form and function.

Vata: Space + Air
Pitta: Fire + Water
Kapha: Water + Earth

With Ayurveda having been discovered thousands of years before technology was invented, Ayurvedic systems, which provide an understanding of certain qualities and how to balance them via counter-balancing energies, were the foundations for healing and living life in balance. The Doshas are simply tools for understanding how to read the body and how to heal it by restoring the balance of appropriate energy. Every ailment or disease is associated with a specific Dosha. By understanding the symptoms, we can decipher the Dosha in dominance and apply these principles to restore balance.

Each of the three Doshas has its own unique set of characteristics. Each have certain qualities in the way that they manifest physically and emotionally; where the Doshas reside within the body and their functions within these domains; and also how they manifest externally, with each Dosha occupying different food groups and influencing certain attributes of our environment. It is these distinct qualities that help us to identify which Dosha is in dominance.

Did you know?

Pitta is made up of Fire + Water, which makes the attributes of Pitta hot, moist, spicy, intense etc., emulating the obvious qualities of fire and water. These qualities can be applied to our physical body and mental state, as well as to food, drinks, lifestyle practices, the weather, times of day, seasons and even the phases of life. Everything, everyone and everywhere has a specific Dosha in dominance, which can help us understand more about ourselves, others and the planet through working with these energies.

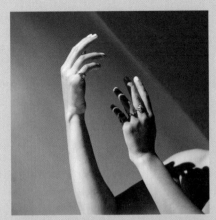
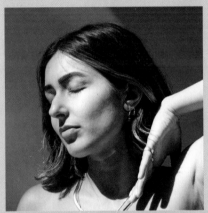
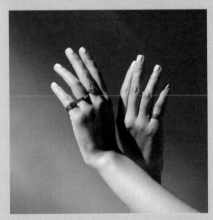

Diving deeper into the Doshas

VATA: SPACE + AIR

These elements make the qualities of Vata cold, dry, light, irregular, rough and brittle. Vata resides in the lower third of the torso – in the colon, pelvis, bladder and reproductive organs, as well as the central nervous system, skeletal system (think bones, nails, teeth, hair) and skin. Issues with digestion, hormone imbalance, UTIs, infertility, joint pain, brittleness, arthritis etc. are associated with Vata aggravations. Vata personalities tend to be social, enthusiastic and creative but can struggle to finish projects and may seem forgetful, airy or anxious if out of balance. The influence of the Air element causes highs and lows in mood, energy, appetite, digestion and sleep. Vata types are petite and thin by nature, they don't require a lot of food and can easily skip a meal. They tend to run cold – often experiencing cold hands and feet; and they suffer from internal and external dryness, with thin hair, dry skin, poor circulation and cracking joints. Vata types are prone to insomnia and anxiety due to their overly active minds. Signs of any of these characteristics in a non-Vata type would signify a Vata aggravation. To reduce the qualities of Vata, a diet and lifestyle consisting of more Kapha qualities would help to ground the flightiness of the Air element, while some Pitta practices could help to add a little heat to get the job done and stay focused.

PITTA: FIRE + WATER

The qualities of Pitta are hot, moist, oily, intense and regular. Pitta's domain is the middle of the trunk, occupying the lower half of the stomach, the liver, gallbladder and small intestine. The Fire element is responsible for breaking down and transforming food into energy, and for all heat within the body. Pitta types are athletic, strong, resilient – they are leaders who require routine and structure. Don't let a Pitta skip a meal! They tend to have strong digestion as the fire burns through almost anything they eat. They run hot, are always on the move and adopt intense lifestyle practices such as vigorous exercise, a demanding career and self-discipline. Pitta aggravations are a result of excess heat in the body, which results in acid reflux, ulcers, fever, diarrhoea, inflammation, strong bodily odours, hair loss, excess sweat and problems with the liver, including impeded detoxification and skin conditions. Feelings of anger, envy, irritability, frustration and impatience are all linked to aggravated Pitta. Once balanced, Pitta types can embrace their natural disposition of strong willpower, courage, confidence, enthusiasm and satisfaction. To restore balance, Kapha practices help to ground and dismantle the heat of Pitta, while Vata can dry out excessive moisture.

KAPHA: WATER + EARTH

Think of Kapha as the heaviest of the three Doshas, as its deeply earthy roots keep it grounded in stability and endurance. The elements inspire qualities that are oily, heavy, slow, smooth, cold and regular. Kapha resides in the upper third of the torso, in the stomach, lungs and heart. Kapha is the gatekeeper of emotion, stability and mental endurance. Kapha types are heavier set, with big bones and a tendency to weight gain; however, their juiciness makes for plump skin, big lips and eyes, thick, luscious hair and a glowing complexion. Kapha types age gracefully and are renowned healers, as they operate from the heart. Kaphas feel the cold and can be weighed down by their emotions, enticing them to overeat and become stagnant; once balanced, though, they possess mental endurance and can be very compassionate. Kapha is responsible for bodily fluids and secretions, and provides lubrication to the joints and moisture to the skin. Excess Kapha can manifest as mucus, congestion, problems with the lungs such as coughs and pneumonia, heart disease and obesity, growths such as cysts and tumours, as well as depression. Kapha is balanced well with Pitta in cases of fatigue, as the fire stimulates action, and Vata provides the balance to dry out excess moisture and reduce growths.

Did you know?

If someone is experiencing hot fever and excessive sweating (Fire + Water attributes) we can recognise that they have a Pitta aggravation (Pitta being Fire + Water), so these symptoms would be pacified by using cooling energies such as bitter greens like mint and coriander (cilantro) (which are cooling by nature), coconut water and cold compresses to 'put out the fire'.

EXPLORING THE DOSHAS

	Vata (Air)	Pitta (Fire)	Kapha (Earth)
Attributes	Cold, dry, light, irregular, rough and brittle	Hot, moist, oily, intense and regular	Cold, oily, smooth, regular, heavy and slow
Physical	Petite, small frame, small features (thin lips, small eyes, discrete nose/jaw), thin skin, thin hair, minimal body hair	Strong, athletic, muscle definition; pronounced features such as strong bones; often red-headed or blonde with fair/reddish skin	Big boned, thick moist skin, plumpness (lips, skin, body), thick, dark hair and round features such as big eyes
Strengths	Social, creative, outgoing, friendly	Leader, gets the job done, accomplished	Compassionate, nurturing, healer
Weaknesses	Anxious, struggles to finish projects, overactive mind, insomnia	Jealous, competitive, bossy, over-stimulated, stressed	Emotional, lethargic, holds a grudge, unmotivated
Foods rich in this Dosha	Crackers, crisps, plain toast, popcorn, raw foods, beans, cruciferous vegetables	Spicy, salty, processed foods, sour foods, pungent foods, chillies, stimulants	Sweets (candy), cakes, pastries, dessert, root vegetables, grains, fats, oils
Lifestyle	Social, active, fun	Intense, action-based	Slow and steady
Physical aggravations	Dry skin, brittle nails, hair shedding, cracking joints, aching pain, toothache, gas and bloating, constipation, period pain, ageing	Fever, excess sweat/body odour, hair loss, reflux, ulcers, liver conditions, skin conditions, allergies, diarrhoea, burning sensations	Excess moisture/secretions in the eyes, ears, sinuses and lungs; growths, cysts, tumours, oedema, heart disease, obesity
Emotional aggravations	Sensitive, forgetful, anxious, distracted, feeling ungrounded	Angry, hot-headed, impulsive, envious, feeling aggressive	Depressed, fatigued, lazy, lethargic, feeling stuck
Balance with	Pitta for action Kapha for grounding	Vata for drying Kapha for slowing down	Vata for reducing Pitta for action

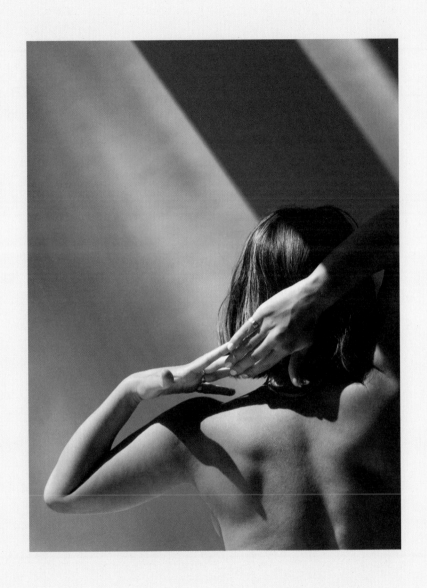

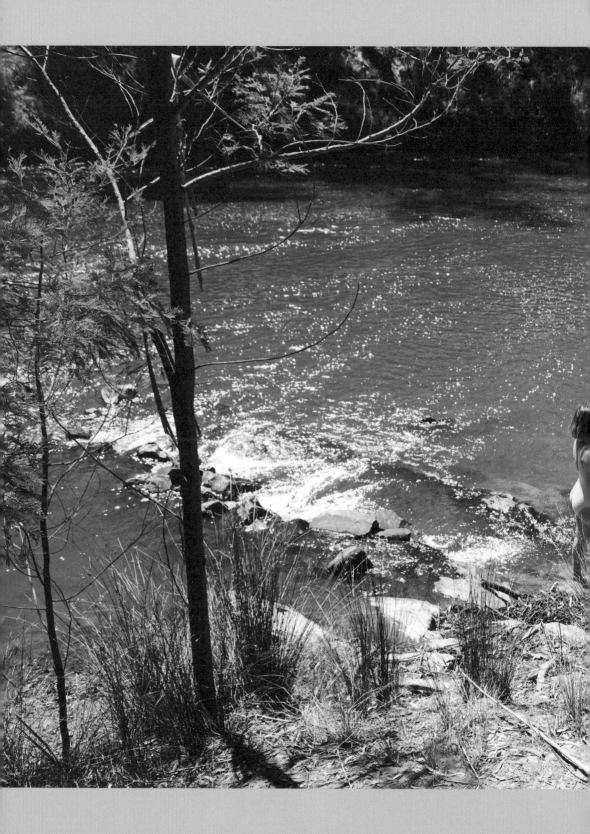

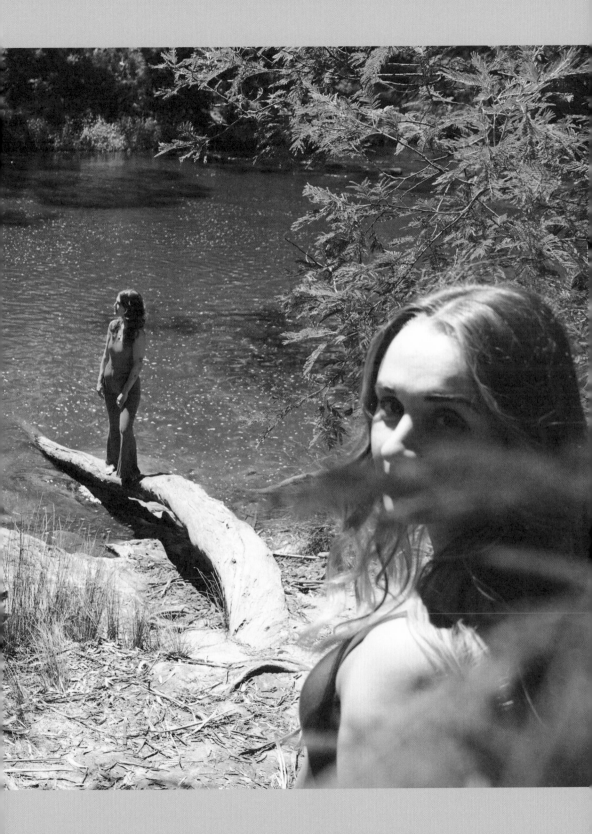

Balancing the Doshas

The secret to understanding Ayurveda is through learning the subtle energies and qualities of the Doshas. Ayurveda recognises three basic types of energy, known as the Three Doshas (Vata, Pitta and Kapha), which are present in everyone and everything.

The process of restoring balance:

Addressing the problem

o   If you are experiencing heaviness, fatigue and lethargy, this indicates that the Kapha Dosha is aggravated. Kapha has Earth energy, so it is heavy, deeply rooted and stagnant.

Finding the balance

o   The opposite of Kapha is to be light, airy and spacious – which are the attributes of Vata (Air). You can add more Vata qualities to your life to lift the stagnation – such as being outdoors (with the wind on your skin), throwing yourself into a creative project, joining a community group, socialising, doing something spontaneous, travelling, and consuming more Vata-rich foods, which are light and uplifting, such as light soups, cruciferous vegetables, healthy salads etc.

This is an extremely powerful method for fully connecting with your body so you can navigate your way through life armed with the tools to restore balance whenever and wherever you are.

Simplicity and logic are key to understanding the attributes of the Doshas. If you are able to look at the Dosha qualities and make sense of them, you will find the answer you're looking for. When getting acquainted with the elements, try to think about what their attributes would look like. The element of Water, for example, would have to be linked to liquid-like properties within the body such as congestion, mucus, secretions, fluid retention and swelling – all qualities that are largely made of water. Once you recognise the element associated with what you are experiencing, you can add the counter-balancing elements to restore balance, so in this case you would add some Fire to your diet and lifestyle to burn off the Water element.

Before the introduction of medical testing, Ayurvedic practitioners would analyse the symptoms of a patient and apply the logic of the Doshas to their diet and lifestyle activities to treat the disease and restore balance. The equation is simple. We look at the innate constitution of a person (which is where harmony lives), then we look at their symptoms and define the aggravated Dosha, then work with the counter-balancing elements to restore homeostasis (balance).

No matter what the disease or health concern we are facing, we can always apply this logic to restore balance. This is a powerful tool for working with your own body on a daily basis to ensure you are always accessing optimum levels of vitality and are able to free yourself from restrictive health boundaries.

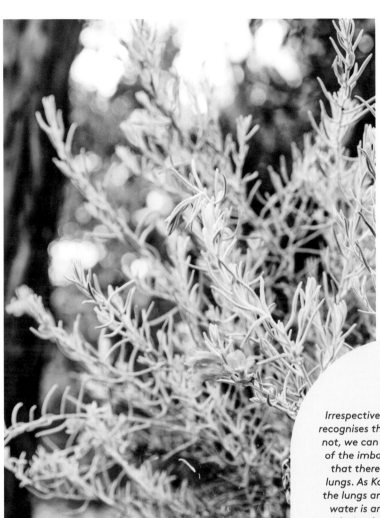

Did you know?

Irrespective of whether Ayurveda recognises the term 'pneumonia' or not, we can look at the symptoms of the imbalance and distinguish that there is excess fluid in the lungs. As Kapha resides largely in the lungs and, as indicated, fluid/water is an attribute of Kapha, it's simple to see that a Kapha aggravation is at play. We would then use the opposing qualities of Air, or Vata, to dry out the excess fluid. All Kapha-aggravating foods, which perpetuate the production of bodily fluids, would be eliminated from the diet (such as oils, fats, sugar and heavy foods). These would be replaced with drying foods to absorb and dry out the liquid in the lungs.

Understanding your constitution

Creating an intimate relationship with yourself is an integral part of infusing the knowledge of Ayurveda into your life. The closer you are to yourself, the deeper your practice, understanding and intuition will become. By uncovering your innate constitution, or Dosha, you will discover more about yourself than ever before.

It's important to understand the difference between your innate constitution (Prakriti) and your current imbalances (Vikriti). Your constitution is determined at your time of conception. Much like your DNA, this establishes all of the qualities that are destined to make you uniquely you. Keeping in mind that we are all made up of varying quantities of all three Doshas, we are often dominated by one or two Doshas that contribute to our strongest attributes from birth. Over time, through exposure to our parents, friends, peers, teachers, media, culture, nature, our environment, and our diet and lifestyle behaviours, we will begin to see fluctuations of other elements appearing in what we believe to be our constitution.

As each Dosha has a colourful and diverse range of attributes, strengths and 'weaknesses', knowing your Dosha can help you accept certain elements about yourself that you may have been struggling with your whole life. Fully embracing your complete essence and realising the strengths that you embody may come as a result of what you have previously considered weaknesses. Once you understand the qualities of your constitution, you can begin to experiment with diet, lifestyle and self-care practices that are specifically designed to uplift your spirit and provide you with support to carry you through some of the more challenging aspects of your mind/body type.

Did you know?

A child who is born with a small frame, seen as 'skinny', very active and social would be considered a Vata type, but if this child is exposed to domestic violence, social isolation, abuse or any range of external factors that could cause depression, we may see the child begin to overeat as a coping mechanism and they may retreat from their otherwise social lifestyle as they battle their internal demons. Later in life, the child could become overweight, shy and likely to keep to themselves – they may then be classified as a Kapha type when in actuality they are a Vata type with a Kapha aggravation.

WHICH DOSHA ARE YOU?

To identify your innate constitution, it's best to look at your characteristics as a child.

o Vata children are thin, active, social, creative, friendly and natural performers. They are fussy eaters and can happily go without big meals.

o Pitta children are leaders – teaching other kids how to play the game and keeping score. They are lean and have muscle definition, and it's hard for them to sit still. They are strong eaters.

o Kapha children are plump, sweet, sensitive, shy, clingy and tend to want to stick with their parents or to be on their own. They love mealtime, snacking and anything sweet.

Which of these types resonates with you? This may hold the answer to your innate constitution.

Our Vikriti reflects the Dosha that is in dominance at the present moment. This is really the most important Dosha to work with, as we need to reduce any aggravations in order to restore balance. If you are a Vata type with a Kapha aggravation, we are going to focus on pacifying Kapha rather than treating you solely as a Vata type. Typically Ayurvedic practitioners prescribe a Kapha-rich diet for a Vata person, as it balances the needs of Vata, but in this case we are actually going to introduce more Pitta and Vata foods to reduce the excess of Kapha. If we were just to treat this person as a Vata type and give them a Kapha-rich diet, we would be fuelling the Kapha aggravation. So it's most important to identify the Dosha that is dominating the skin, body, mind or lifestyle and reduce its qualities first in order for balance to be properly restored.

Did you know?

As humans, the element of Earth dominates our bones, Water governs our bodily fluids, Fire imparts the heat that transforms and powers our digestion, and Air provides the oxygen that is the very basis of our existence. Flowers and plants grow from soil and their roots keep them deeply grounded in the Earth element. Birds possess much more of the Air + Space elements, as their lightness and feathers create a buoyancy that allows them to soar the skies above. Regardless of which of these great elements are dominant, each of us possesses the qualities of all five, just in varying quantities. This specific makeup gives a flair to our uniqueness as a species and as individuals. Each person has their own signature, made up of each element; some may possess more Fire, others more Earth, forming the basis of their Dosha, and equating to their unique constitution.

FINDING THE BALANCE

Every aspect of Ayurveda always comes back to finding and restoring balance. It's important to recognise that every negative has a positive and that by working with these polarities we can begin to appreciate all of the elements that form our own unique blueprint of qualities and that fuel the passions of our life and the story we will one day tell.

As a Vata type:

o **Mentally** you may struggle with completing projects. But, on the other hand, it is your constant stream of creativity that fuels a never-ending list of ideas and dreams. Vata types work well with Pitta types to see ideas come to fruition.

o **Socially** you may find it hard to walk down the street without having to stop and say hello to a number of people, but it is your ability to connect with others that creates your ever-expanding social network.

o **Physically** you may have wished for longer, thicker hair and more radiant skin but it is the Air element within you that keeps you light on your feet and free from the shackles of weight gain.

o **Your diet and skincare regime** will be focused on adding more moisture to balance the qualities of Air through the use of oils, fats and earthy foods (Kapha), as well as heat to ignite your internal fire and move things along (Pitta).

o **Your lifestyle** will centre around grounding the airiness of Vata through slowing down, going inward, connecting with yourself, having some alone time, journalling and meditating.

As a Pitta type:

o **Mentally** you may feel an immense amount of internal pressure to set milestones and achieve goals, but it is this drive that makes you a natural-born leader who will achieve great success in life. If you struggle to get out of your head and into a creative space, partner up with a Vata type to ignite the creative juices.

o **Socially** you don't have time for idle chit-chat and like to have your social interactions pre-planned to suit your busy schedule; it is this routine that allows you to accomplish a great sense of self-discipline and mastery.

o **Physically** you have a strong frame and may have fantasised over a more petite or curvaceous figure but the Fire element that builds you up is also the reason for your hearty digestion, endurance and physical stamina.

o **Your diet and skincare regime** will be centred around cooling the fire, as you are quick to heat up and need the elements of Vata to absorb excess moisture and Kapha to calm the blaze.

o **Your lifestyle** will focus on releasing your fiery internal conflict and goal-orientated mental disposition with the introduction of more spontaneity, social interaction and relaxation.

As a Kapha type:

o **Mentally** you are weighed down by your emotions and can become lethargic as a result but it is your deeply sensitive empathy that makes you an amazing caregiver, friend, partner, parent and teacher.

o **Socially** you may carry the weight of the world on your shoulders. People often come to you for advice and you may get stuck carrying the load, but with some healthy boundaries, you can become a great healer and support system for yourself and those you care about.

o **Physically** you are prone to weight gain and often struggle to stay in shape but these qualities also give lustre to your skin, eyes, hair and nails and will ensure you age gracefully, as your skin retains moisture and your tissues have an endless stream of nourishment.

o **Your diet and skincare regime** is the least demanding of all. Your body holds a well of nutrition and little is required from you other than avoiding Kapha-aggravating foods such as sweets (candy) and fats in excess.

o **Your lifestyle** will be centred around movement and getting you motivated to achieve all of the wonderful things in your destiny. Socialising and breaking out of your comfort zone are the best ways to find your inner voice.

MOTHER NATURE + THE SEASONS

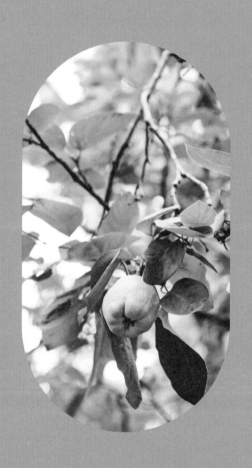

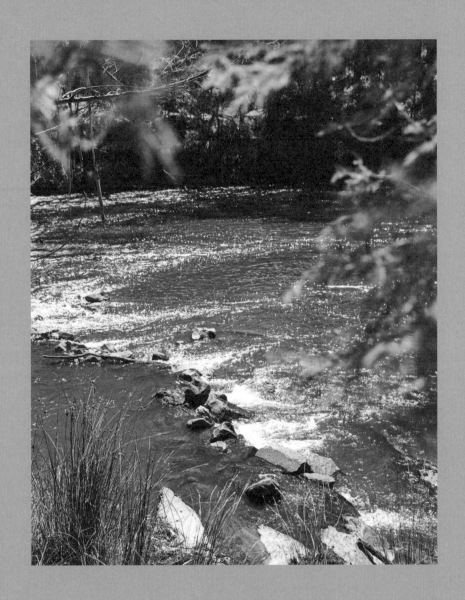

3

Understanding our environment + the elements
(Pancha Maha Bhutas)

ETHER · AIR · FIRE · WATER · EARTH

We are a reflection of the world we live in. We share a common thread with everything that surrounds us, including other people, animals, plants, flowers, even colours, sounds and inanimate objects. This is because we are all made up of a unique combination of the same things. Basically, there are only five key ingredients – the Five Great Elements (Pancha Maha Bhutas) of Space, Air, Fire, Water and Earth – that comprise everything that exists here on earth, yet the varying quantities of each of these ingredients largely affect the final product.

As we are made up of the same five elements as everything that surrounds us, it makes sense that these elements are all that is necessary to sustain life. As creatures of planet earth, our environment provides us with everything we need to survive. It is what it was designed to do and it has done so for millions of years. Anything outside of what is naturally abundant in our habitat is likely to add stress to the body as our internal forces try to comprehend this other-worldly matter. We are made of the Five Elements and we survive off the Five Elements. To have a balanced diet, providing all the nutrition we require, all we need is food made up of these elements. Food, beauty and household products, and other products such as pharmaceuticals, that have been produced out

of synthetic (unnatural) ingredients – including artificial colours, flavours, preservatives, chemicals, foods that have been bleached, sprayed, genetically modified or those that have been processed/altered from their original form – are all indigestible to the human body. Food is energy; it should be natural, come from the earth, and contain the same elements we possess, so that it is able to replenish and revitalise our life force.

To live a life as nature intended is to live symbiotically with the land. Before humankind evolved to where we are today, we treated the planet as we would our own home – please let that sink in for a minute. Before the advent of construction and the industrial revolution, the earth was all we had. She offered shelter, somewhere to rest our weary head, to cook our loving meals and bathe away the day, everything we needed all within her earthly bounty. She would provide and in return we would respect, honour and cherish her. As humans, we actually didn't have a large role to play in the function of the planet other than to allow it to do what it was designed to do. Left in harmony, the trees clean the air; the insects, plants and animals sustain the food chain; the rain, rivers and streams water the garden; the sun feeds the plants; the moon creates cycles and controls the

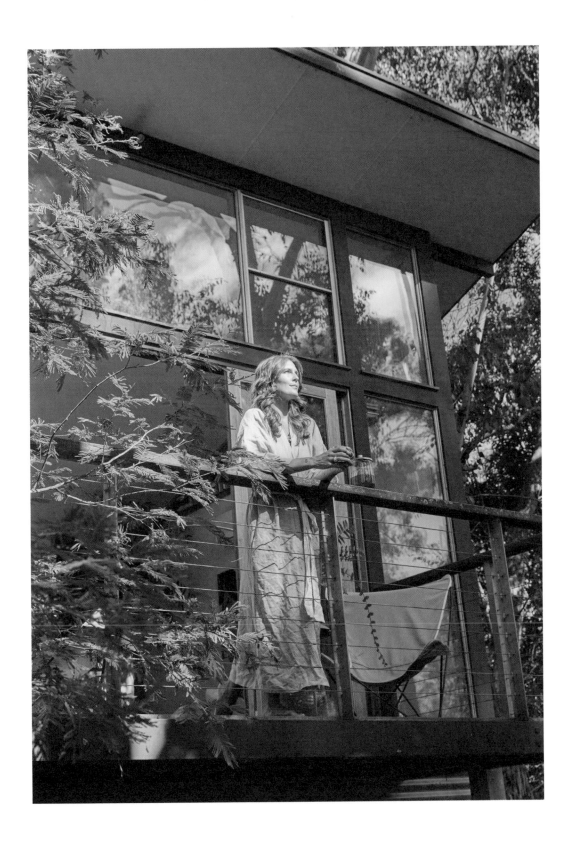

ocean – everything is perfect. Every single thing has a place and a purpose. When this perfect balance is overturned, problems arise. Humans have played a devastating role in the destruction of this perfect harmony. By cutting down trees, contaminating waterways, engaging in industrial farming, polluting the air and pillaging and over-developing rural land, we are restricting the symbiotic nature of the earth. Everything we do has an impact, and we are beginning to realise the detrimental effects of our actions.

The more the earth suffers and is hindered from creating what we need to survive, the bigger the problem becomes. As we build up and out, we reduce the opportunity for local farming and foraging, instead relying on international trade, which really perpetuates the problem, as we begin to consume foods that are not in season and don't support the conditions we encounter in our local environment.

Eating cooling summer fruits that are high in sugar, such as watermelon, during winter is counter-intuitive to the needs of our body, which is why you won't find it growing in winter. Mother Nature knows exactly what we need and when we need it, and she provides just that. We should be eating foods that are grown locally and picked fresh to preserve their life force. As there are a multitude of different climates all across the world, existing simultaneously but with unique qualities, it's important to work within your natural habitat. When the weather is warm, your environment will provide cooling fruits and plants that complement the needs of your surrounding elements. When the weather cools, root vegetables and heating plants will bloom to add some bulk and fire to your diet to compensate for the lack of warmth. International trade also contributes largely to air and water pollution, further exaggerating the problem of our modern way of living.

Our environment is our natural living habitat, the provider of everything we need to survive and prosper. Every manufactured product is a replication of something natural – or has nature as its roots. The problem is that we take what Mother Nature has so beautifully formulated for us, then manipulate, process and totally reshape the original source into something that our body does not have the intelligence or programming to process. Our environment should always be the inspiration for how we live our lives on a daily basis.

Did you know?

As humans, the element of Earth dominates our bones, Water governs our bodily fluids, Fire imparts the heat that transforms and powers our digestion, and Air provides the oxygen that is the very basis of our existence. Flowers and plants grow from soil and their roots keep them deeply grounded in the Earth element. Birds possess much more of the Air + Space elements, as their lightness and feathers create a buoyancy that allows them to soar the skies above. Regardless of which of these great elements are dominant, each of us possesses the qualities of all five, just in varying quantities. This specific makeup gives a flair to our uniqueness as a species and as individuals. Each person has their own signature, made up of each element; some may possess more Fire, others more Earth, forming the basis of their Dosha, and equating to their unique constitution.

In a spiritual sense, the earth is our home and we are designed to be surrounded by the beauty that abounds. To bask in the warmth of the morning sun, to lose ourselves in the aroma of wildflowers, to pause as we listen to the sounds of birds singing, to dive into the refreshing elixir of a springwater creek, to elevate the senses through a refreshing bounty of hand-foraged berries. These are the moments that make our soul sing. These are the practices that bring our body, mind and spirit back into alignment, that reconnect us with Mother Nature, our true home, and create a poetic resonance between our soul and our senses.

The seasons

Throughout the year, each of the Doshas occupies certain seasons, largely reflecting the dominant elements in our environment. With this knowledge, we can cultivate a lifestyle that accommodates these mighty forces so that we can live in unison with our surroundings, allowing nature to guide us through each phase. Classically, Ayurveda recognises six seasons, including monsoon and drought periods, but for simplicity, we will focus on the four main seasons we are more accustomed to.

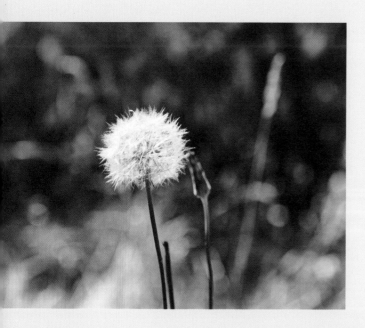

Ayurveda identifies the unique form and function of each of the seasons, in which nature expresses itself as a living, breathing entity.

It is important to honour the seasons and work with them as a force of nature, rather than to force against nature, so that you can move through the year with grace and fluidity, performing shifts in energy, diet and lifestyle practices at the turn of each season.

Each season pacifies or ignites certain energies within us, meaning that our bodies can be thrown out of balance if we don't take the correct measures to adapt.

SPRING (KAPHA/PITTA)

Spring is a time of new beginnings. Nature bounds back to life as flowers bloom, birds sing, and both people and animals arise from slumber. Naturally the sun inspires more energy and creation as everything begins to switch on and activate. This is a potent time for cleansing and bringing ideas to life. Adversely, the excess Water element of Kapha season can result in allergies and excess mucus; cleansing and a Vata diet is useful for pacifying these symptoms.

SUMMER (PITTA)

Summer is an intoxicating time of excess heat as the Fire element burns through the scorching months. With Pitta at an all-time high, it is best to avoid excessively vigorous exercise and instead adopt a mellow, cooling lifestyle to extinguish the fire, otherwise excess heat provokes inflammation and liver conditions, and is known to cause breakouts, rashes or skin irritations such as acne, psoriasis and eczema. You may find your digestion suffers during this time of year as it battles with excess heat,

so it's important to support your digestive fire/metabolism (Agni).

AUTUMN (VATA)

Autumn celebrates the end of long, hot summer days as the Air element drives in wind and recalibrates the tune to accommodate more mild temperatures. Vata season is particularly drying, both internally and externally, so it's important to nourish the body and skin with warming oils and to introduce additional fibre to your diet. During autumn we are prone to hair shedding, flaky skin and constipation along with indecisiveness and anxiety, so don't be alarmed when you experience these symptoms, but do what you can to support yourself through this process with the help of a grounding Kapha diet and lifestyle.

WINTER (VATA/KAPHA)

Winter provides the perfect antidote to a long, hot summer of action and intensity. It is a time for reflection, rest and respite. It embodies qualities of peace and harmony, but the Earth element can also trigger sensations of heaviness, fatigue and lethargy, and can leave you feeling isolated, alone and even depressed if not balanced. Kapha season promotes endurance, memory (this is a great time to take a course), meditation, introspection and self-healing. With our digestive fire at its strongest point throughout the year, now is the time to indulge in heavier, grounding meals, such as root vegetables, soups, stews and hearty curries – even some sweet foods. As we are eating more, it's also important to move more to lift stagnant energy through vigorous exercise and activity.

Seasonal rituals

The process of honouring the cycles of the year is known as Ritucharya. Ritu means 'season' and charya means 'to follow'.

As we are creatures who are part of an entire ecosystem that fluctuates vastly to support the ever-changing needs of the earth as a whole, all we can effectively control is the choices we make to exist within the natural world.

Consciously choosing to connect with nature strengthens our alignment to the cosmic forces at play, allowing us to access a deeper relationship with the Elements and our natural world.

Our intuition naturally gravitates towards practices that are complementary to our environment, such as indulging in warming soups and stews during winter, or diving into a fresh watermelon in the summer, but the influence of modern inventions such as air-conditioning and heating can throw our innate sensitivities off balance. By coming back to our awareness of the seasons and allowing our intuition to be our guide, we have a better chance of accessing year-round balance.

Did you know?

Ayurveda adopts the philosophy that 'like increases like', meaning that during Pitta season, for example, the qualities of Pitta are magnified. Anyone with a Pitta constitution, or aggravation, will feel especially hot, agitated and fired up during Pitta season, so it's even more important to invest in Pitta-pacifying diet and lifestyle practices to 'put out the fire'.

A Vata person may find their skin especially dry and experience excess hair shedding during autumn and early winter as Vata energy is at play in the environment, which comes with the attributes of dryness and airiness.

A Kapha type who has a tendency towards depression may feel burdened with feelings of heaviness during late winter/spring when the Earth element dominates.

Be mindful of your constitution and be aware of when this Dosha comes into dominance through the year so you can work to find balance. By making choices that neutralise the effects of each season, you can maintain your internal sense of equilibrium throughout the year.

HONOURING THE SEASONS

Season	Dominant Dosha	Qualities	Do	Avoid
Spring	Kapha/Pitta	Excess Water element (rain), causing swelling, water retention, allergies, congestion, lethargy and discomfort	Movement, yoga, pranayama (breathing exercises), meditation, cleanse Kapha	Stagnation, heavy food
Summer	Pitta	Excess Fire element (heat), causing skin irritations, weak digestion, perspiration, liver conditions and irritability	Cooling activities like swimming, meditation, slow walks, slowing down, staying cool; consume a cooling diet	Increasing the heart rate, vigorous exercise, excessive activity, heating and stimulating diet
Autumn	Vata	Excess Air element (wind), causing dryness, constipation, flaky skin, hair shedding, insomnia, anxiety and brain fog	Slow down, keep warm and nourished; eat warming, soothing and easily digestible meals	Being overly social, instead begin to withdraw and go inward; avoid exposure to wind
Winter	Vata/Kapha	Excess Air and Water elements, causing dryness, hair shedding, brittleness, cracking joints, fragility, lethargy and withdrawal	Rest, hibernate, recuperate, meditate, be creative; eat warming, nourishing meals	Stagnation; this is a time for movement to burn off the extra food required in winter

THE ART
OF LIVING

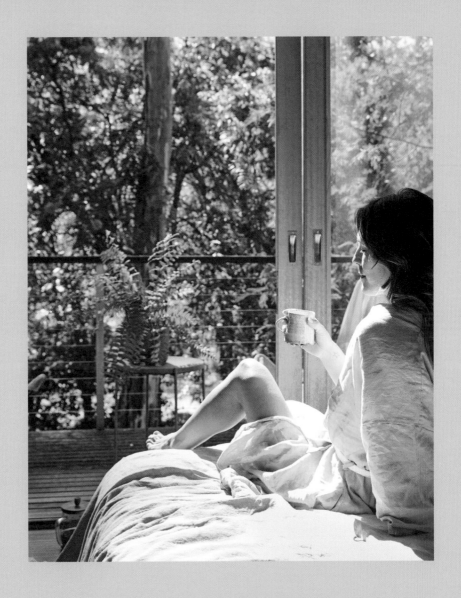

4

Dosha clock – crafting your day

Every day is an opportunity to create the life we long to live and the legacy we wish to leave, for our life to be an expression of our soul. We craft our days, our weeks and our months and have the power to do this in a way that either does or does not serve our highest self.

The Dosha Clock deciphers the optimum times to eat, sleep, work, create, socialise, exercise and rest in alignment with the energy of the natural world and how these activities are best supported by our environment and the elements. Each of the three Doshas comes into dominance twice throughout the day, at the same time in the AM and PM but with slightly different functions based on the masculine energy of the sun and the feminine energy of the moon. When a Dosha is in dominance, we always use the qualities of the opposite Dosha to restore balance.

THE DOSHA CLOCK

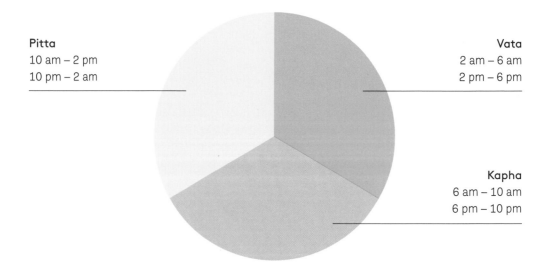

Pitta
10 am – 2 pm
10 pm – 2 am

Vata
2 am – 6 am
2 pm – 6 pm

Kapha
6 am – 10 am
6 pm – 10 pm

THE DOSHA CLOCK

Time	Dominant Dosha	Do	Avoid
2 am – 6 am	Vata	Sleep: this is when your body begins to reboot for the day; it's healthy to wake up any time after 4 am if your body is in a balanced state and you have had enough sleep; this is the ideal time for meditation	Being awake during this time; you may rise between 4 am and 6 am to get the most out of your day and ensure you are ready for sleep again in the evening when the sun goes down
6 am – 10 am	Kapha	Wake up, meditate, practise yoga and pranayama (breathing exercises), exercise, nourish Rasa (see page 133), eat breakfast, cleanse/bathe, study	Sleeping through this window, as you will fall into a very deep Kapha sleep, leaving you excessively tired; avoid heavy meals
10 am – 2 pm	Pitta	Get chores, jobs and tasks done, prepare and consume your largest meal of the day	Intense exercise, direct sunlight, stressful situations, confrontation, anything excessively 'heating'
2 pm – 6 pm	Vata	Socialise, problem solve, get creative and crafty	Windy or cold environments, anything too drying; heavy meals
6 pm – 10 pm	Kapha	Unwind, read, practise self-care and prepare yourself for sleep, switch from artificial light to candles and amber light	Devices and any forms of artificial light or stimulation; heavy meals
10 pm – 2 am	Pitta	Sleep: this is when most of your digestion occurs and your body works on deep healing; if you are awake at this time, your energy will be redirected into staying awake, making you overstimulated, and you will not have the chance to heal and repair as you would if you were sleeping	Staying awake

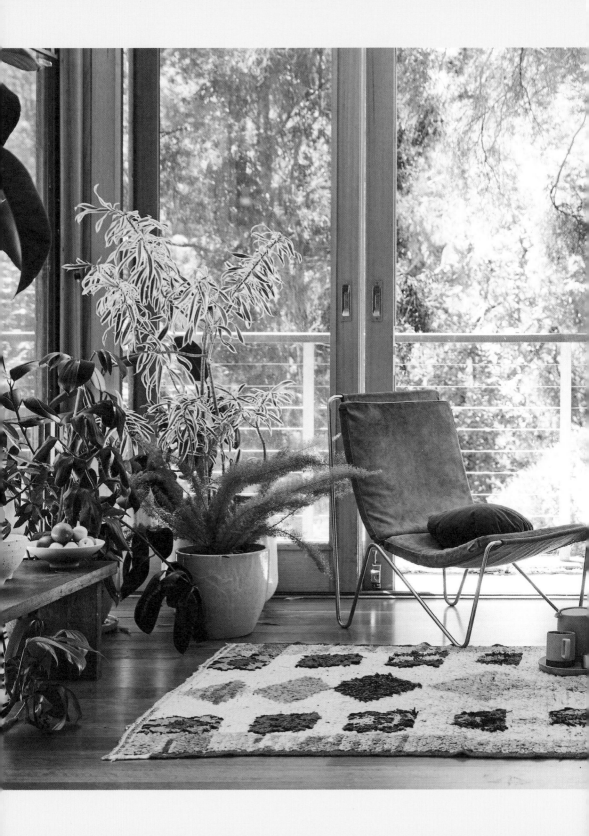

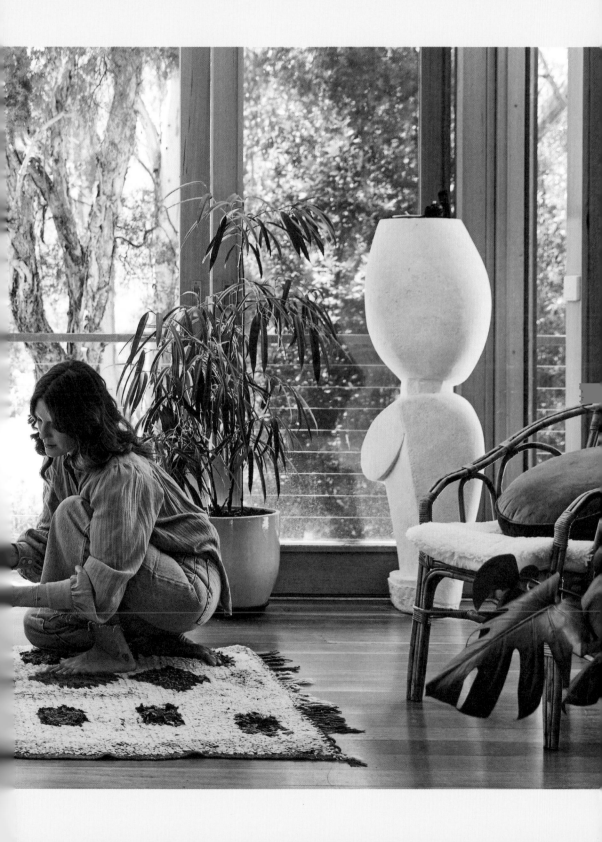

Ritual

As a holistic lifestyle, Ayurveda offers a treasure trove of rituals to support your ever-changing needs in alignment with the fluidity of nature and the shifts in seasons. These ancient practices were designed to enhance the vitality of life and impart a form of sensuality into your experiences.

They intensify your opportunity for ultimate health and wellbeing as rituals that support the body's detoxification processes, boost the immune system, improve physical wellbeing, calm the mind, and inspire deep sleep and a positive outlook.

Two terms that come into play when cultivating dedication to your daily rituals are Sadhana and Tapas. Anything that is practised with awareness, discipline and the intention of spiritual growth can be considered Sadhana – from preparing your meals through to meditation. This practice requires a surrendering of the ego in order to access the full potential of mindfulness. Tapas involves the power associated with the confidence to shake off any dispelling beliefs you may have about yourself, your potential or the reasoning behind your action. In Sanskrit, Tapas means 'to heat or burn up', referring to the way discipline burns off the space for negative self-talk and self-imposed limitations. These are important philosophies to keep in mind when crafting your schedule, as change often comes with resistance. Remember that you are in control and that these rituals are ultimately here to improve and revitalise your life.

You may be ready to dive in completely, or you may like to take a slower approach and begin to integrate the rituals that resonate with you the most. It's about crafting a practice that aligns with your goals and complements your schedule, without tipping the boat too far over. The first step towards approaching this way of living involves deeply connecting the subconscious and conscious mind so that you can cultivate intention and awareness in everything you do. This allows your body to connect fully with each experience, magnifying the effect and allowing you to absorb the true essence of what you're feeling. By expressing gratitude for the joy you receive as a result of your practices, you will further nurture the deepest layers of your being and allow the benefits to become more and more potent.

Begin experimenting with the rituals that sing out to you and see if you can find a way to integrate them into your daily life. The deeper your love affair with these humbling practices grows, the further they will be cemented into your psyche.

AYURVEDIC DAILY RITUALS

Far from the madding modern world of fast-paced action and go go go, Ayurveda offers a much slower approach to beginning the day so that we can move forward with a clear mind and nourished body as a daily benchmark. Dinacharya is the Sanskrit term for 'daily rituals' that help to support a life of optimal wellness through routine, detoxification and nourishment. This practice is at the heart of the Ayurvedic lifestyle and is the backbone that enables health to thrive.

Dinacharya is one of the most powerful tools for regaining control over your life, through ensuring that each and every day includes rituals that support and nourish you. Having structure in your day gives you purpose and guidance. This is especially grounding for anyone suffering from mental health issues, depression or anxiety. When you have a routine in place, you know what you have to do and when it has to be done. This alleviates the vastness of ideas on how to begin your day, which can be overwhelming at times.

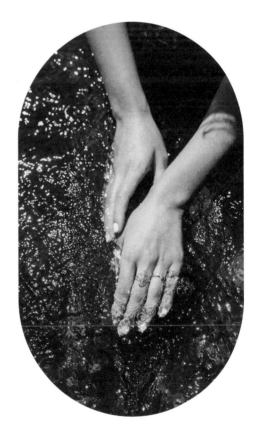

The discipline of routine and repetition is more beneficial than trying to squeeze in little bits of everything on any given day, so if you're time poor, start with setting a time of day you'd like to wake up, then introduce each practice one at a time. Keep in mind that Ayurveda honours the early hours of the morning, as the essence of calmness and tranquillity imbibes the energy before the world begins to kick into action. This is a potent time for stillness, clarity, healing and rewiring neural pathways that form our patterns. With that in mind, most rituals are done prior to breakfast to set the tone for the day and access a greater sense of inner positivity that you can carry with you.

MORNING RITUALS

1. Rise with the sun

Ideally rise before 6 am, as the Vata elements at this time inspire a sense of lightness and clarity that make it easier to get up, versus Kapha time (6 am – 10 am), which has a much heavier, more dormant energy. Your frame of mind sets the tone for the day, actively choose to begin your day with positive thoughts so that you can carry that energy with you.

2. Eliminate

Eliminate the bladder and bowels to support detoxification, paying attention to any discomfort you may experience, and observing the quality of your eliminations to notice how your meals have been affecting you. After lying horizontal all night, your blood and organs should apply natural pressure to your bowel. Healthy stool should be well formed, medium brown in colour and should float. Urine should be a light yellow colour with no strong odour. Anything outside of this indicates an imbalance in the body that needs to be addressed.

3. Tongue scrape

This is an ancient practice that uses a copper or stainless steel tongue scraper to (painlessly) scrape away bacteria and toxins (Ama) that have been expelled through the tongue overnight as we sleep. It is vital to cleanse this build-up before drinking or eating so we don't recirculate it into our system. Massaging the tongue also awakens and stimulates the vital organs connected to different parts of the tongue, which activates the digestive system.

o   Using a tongue scraper, scrape from the back of your tongue to the front up to seven times, then rinse.

4. Brush your teeth

Do this before eating or drinking also, as the biofilm produced overnight contains bacteria that you don't want riding into your system on the back of your breakfast. Opt for a natural toothpaste that contains antibacterial herbs like anise, cloves, fennel and mint. (See page 92 for Antibacterial toothpaste recipe).

5. Oil pull 'Gandush'

Oils contain many beneficial nutrients that support the strength of our teeth, especially black sesame oil, which is rich in calcium. The daily practice of oil pulling helps to remove plaque and other toxins that can be found in the mouth, while supporting overall oral hygiene and moisturising the gums, resulting in naturally strong, healthy and white teeth. (See page 93 for Oil pulling blend recipe).

6. Drink warm water

Ushapaan is the practice of drinking up to 1 litre of warm water first thing in the morning to lubricate the tissues, aid digestion and detoxification, nourish the skin, support the liver, and provide a healthy amount of hydration for the day. It's important to do this straight after brushing your teeth and 30 minutes before you consume any food so you don't dilute the stomach acids needed for digestion; also avoid cold water, as this dampens Agni (digestive fire).

7. Meditate

Meditation is a way for us to bathe or cleanse the mind, eliminating impurities and purging negative thoughts while rediscovering harmony. Ayurveda regards meditation as the ultimate form of medicine, as the simple practice of stilling the mind allows the body to restore and rejuvenate. No medicine, plant or treatment can compare to the body's innate ability to heal itself. This is programmed into our survival methods and capabilities, but when we are in a state of distress this ability is severely compromised, so by practising meditation we are ultimately providing the body with an opportunity and the support to heal itself. There is no health condition that would not benefit from the practice of meditation. It also contributes to the condition of our physical features, as when we are relaxed, our cells are rejuvenated and we can begin to glow from the inside out.

Meditation is best practised at sunrise, just after waking, to access the 'sleep state' where your conscious mind hasn't completely activated and you are less preoccupied with racing thoughts, or at sunset – it's best to find a time that suits your schedule. It's better to do it at any time rather than not do it at all.

Meditation practice

o Sit in a comfortable position (outside of your bed), close your eyes and focus on taking deep inhalations and exhalations. Listen to your breath leave and enter your body, observe your chest rising and falling, observe any thoughts that may enter your mind and send them away gently, always coming back to your breath. Do this for as little as five minutes per day and you will notice a remarkable difference in your attitude and energy throughout the day, as well as your sleep patterns.

o There are several forms of meditation, including guided meditations, mantra, candle gazing (Trataka) and transcendental, among others. Experiment and find a practice that works for you, but aim to come back to a form of meditation that allows all of your senses to shut off completely (that is, no sound, sight, taste, touch or smell).

8. Massage

At the heart of Ayurvedic daily rituals is the practice of self-massage, known as Abhyanga, which uses warm oil to indulge the senses, balance all Doshas and restore harmony. The word for oil (Sneha) in Sanskrit is translated as 'love', as this form of ritual is the deepest kind of self-love to indulge in. This practice is renowned for promoting longevity, reducing physical and mental fatigue, purifying the entire body, enhancing the complexion through nourishing the skin to make it glow, while also building strength and toning the body.

Massage your body with warm black sesame oil or a crafted oil blend (see page 78) to stimulate circulation; improve the lymphatic system; remove stored toxins and dissolve cellulite; improve skin elasticity and collagen production; maintain breast health and reveal any unwanted blockages; support bone and joint health; heal and prevent injuries; relax the nervous system (reducing stress, anxiety and depression); promote deep sleep; and calm the mind.

Abhyanga practice

o Place a towel on the floor of a warm room and place a small dish of oil beside the towel, so you can dip your hands into it as you go. You may like to heat the oil slightly, either by placing it in an oil burner with a tealight candle underneath or by placing a small jar of oil in a bowl of hot water, being careful not to burn yourself.

o Begin by rubbing your hands together to generate heat, then, starting at the head, use your fingertips to massage the scalp from the base of your hairline to the crown of the head; move to your face and, starting from the forehead, massage along the brows, around the temples, across the cheeks and jaw, working from the centre of the face to the hairline, around and inside the ears, down the neck and shoulders, across the collarbones and around the shoulder joints.

o Hold your hands over your heart and pour loving thoughts into your psyche. Massage over the heart and chest in a clockwise direction. This is particularly nourishing when experiencing heartache or sadness.

o Work your way from under the armpit to the areola (nipple) and around the breast – be gentle and look out for any bumps or causes for concern. Proper lymphatic drainage of the breast is an excellent preventative for breast cancer, and by regularly massaging your breasts you have the best chance of noticing anything at its earliest stage.

o Work clockwise around your stomach, starting from the right hip, upwards to underneath the right rib cage, across to the left rib cage, over the stomach and liver, then down to the left hip. Repeat this path several times, ensuring you work your stomach, liver and intestines. Be gentle moving across the womb/ovaries.

o Move to your left hand and work the pads and the fingers, massaging each joint; work up the arms in long strokes, around the elbows then upwards to the shoulders.

o Repeat on the right.

o Massage your way down the left leg, taking long strokes along the thigh, including the back and lower buttocks. With your leg bent, cup your hand around your kneecap and work in gentle circles around the surrounding tissue and behind. Continue along the shins and calf muscles.

o Move down to the foot and begin massaging the underneath side first; be sure to work the joints of the toes, heel and ankle in circular motions. Massage deeply in between the toes. The feet can handle a lot of pressure and this is where most of our channels begin, so don't hold back here.

o Repeat on the right leg and foot.

o Stand up and work on the buttocks and lower back, moving upwards towards the heart.

Did you know?

Use long strokes on the limbs and circular motions around the joints, always directing the flow back towards the heart to support lymphatic drainage. The lymphatic system doesn't have a pump, so this practice heavily influences your power of detoxification and circulation, which essentially provides fresh oxygen to cells and organs, refreshing and rejuvenating their functionality.

As this practice releases toxins from the skin, it is important to cleanse the oil off within one hour. Avoid this practice during menstruation or while unwell.

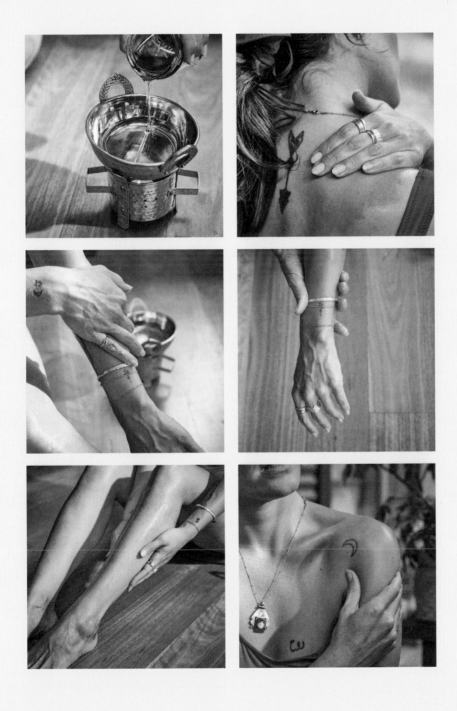

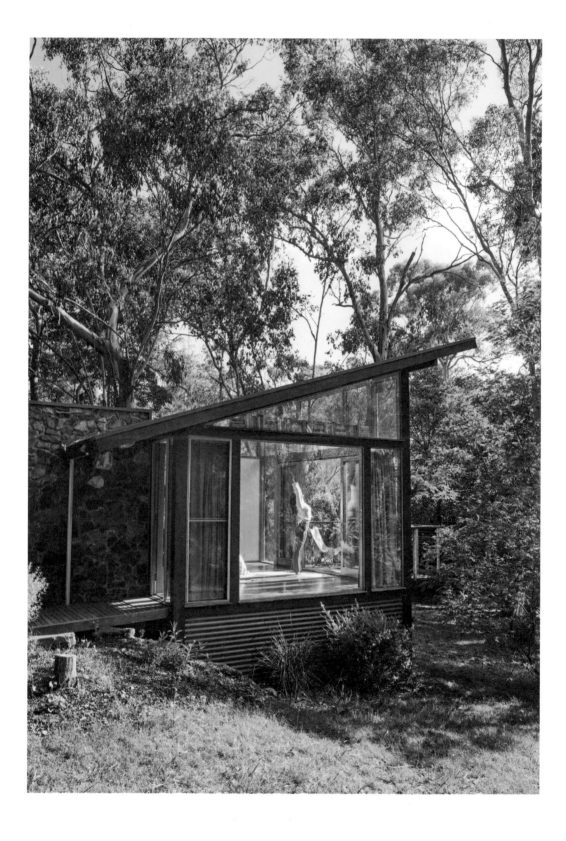

9. Movement

Practise yoga or movement in the morning to counterbalance stagnation and rigidity from sleeping all night. Yoga translates to 'union' in Sanskrit and of all the forms of movement it has the deepest benefits for uniting the body and mind while cultivating a spiritual practice of inner peace and harmony.

o Yoga comes in many forms, from restorative to strengthening. Explore different styles and find a nice mixture of practices that allows you both to build strength (Yang) and relax (Yin), all while cultivating a deeper connection between your body and mind.

o Movement or exercise should be valued as an expression of self-love, with the idea of flexibility (freedom from rigidity later in life), longevity and detoxification at the core of your intentions. Pull yourself back from 'loathing' the idea of exercise; it should never be seen as punishment or a chore – be grateful that you have the opportunity to utilise your body in this way and have fun with it.

Recommended styles of movement for each Dosha:

o **Vata:** Grounding practices such as Hatha and Yin yoga, hot yoga in the cooler months, pilates, long walks or hiking, dance, and some light strength training to build muscle mass. Avoid cooling practices like swimming unless the weather is warm.

o **Pitta:** Cooling practices nearby or in water such as swimming, paddleboarding, canoeing etc., also snow sports such as skiing or ice skating, restorative yoga and slow walks. Avoid competitive and high-intensity sports such as boxing and football etc., as they are likely to aggravate Pitta. You can opt for tennis or more gentle group sports to fulfill your competitive streak.

o **Kapha:** Practices to get you moving and work up a sweat such as power walking, dance, hot yoga, Vinyasa yoga, pilates, and some socially competitive sports like tennis, netball, volleyball etc. to get you out of your comfort zone.

10. Cleanse

Cleanse your body with natural products. Our skin is our largest organ and everything that comes into contact with it enters our bloodstream. Less is more in terms of using different products and soaps; we want our skin to have a chance to produce its own oils and absorb the ones we add to it, so resist the temptation to scrub your body daily. Keep the temperature of your shower as low as you can handle. Hot water burns the skin, causing dehydration, which definitely speeds up the ageing process. Cold showers are ideal during summer and enliven the senses. Warm showers are useful for removing dirt and bacteria, but try not to overdo it. Experiment with making your own natural self-care products to provide the most nutrition to your skin while avoiding harsh chemicals.

As is the mind, so is the body.

Perhaps one of the most fundamental aspects of Ayurveda is the intrinsic relationship between the mind and body. Modern science has now uncovered what Ayurveda has known for thousands of years – there is a direct connection between the brain and the body, and emotion has an instant effect on the form and function of our organs, bodily tissues and just about every process the body performs on a daily basis.

This is how it works – your sense organs (eyes, ears, nose, tongue, skin) respond to elements or triggers in your environment. The brain then converts this emotion into an action and that action usually has a positive or negative effect on the body through the release of certain hormones. If the body senses anger/stress/danger, it will produce the hormone cortisol, which is useful for getting out of tricky situations, but at the same time it also suppresses the immune system in order to preserve strength for survival. Surgeons utilise the immune-suppressing qualities of cortisol when performing organ transplants, injecting the patient with cortisol to prevent the immune system from rejecting the foreign organ. So, clearly, if we are constantly in a state of stress, our immune system can become severely compromised. On the other hand, if we experience feelings of joy/love/happiness, we release hormones like serotonin, dopamine and oxytocin, and endorphins, which allow the body to relax and access a state of bliss. This ultimately inspires deep rest, healing and other rejuvenating processes that contribute to graceful ageing, strong immunity, long-term health and a calm state of mind.

If you look at the mind as the control centre for the entire body, it makes absolute sense to recognise the link between negative emotion and disease. Studies have monitored the direct link between the brain and the effect that stress or negative emotion has on the liver – showing an instant contraction and contortion of the liver when exposed to stress. This distortion prevents the liver from conducting its usual processes of cleansing and detoxifying (among many other functions). So you can imagine that after experiencing this for a long period of time, the body would slowly begin to suffer the consequences of insufficient organ function. The same happens in the gut. The gut, known as the 'second brain', reacts to mental activity and actually experiences fluctuations in emotions alongside the mind. This is where terms like 'gut feeling' or 'kicked in the guts' come from. Stress can literally halt gut function entirely and, as a result, a plethora of digestive issues can arise, such as IBS, constipation, diarrhoea etc., which then go on to cause accumulative disorders, allergies, skin conditions etc. When our organs aren't given the opportunity to do what they need to do, we begin to see the signs in our skin, hair, teeth, nails, all over

– this is our body telling us something isn't functioning properly and we need to heal.

With the knowledge and understanding that disease is very much triggered by the brain as a reaction to our emotional experiences, or that 'disease begins in the mind', Ayurveda prescribes mental health as the priority and basic foundation for wellbeing. Where the thoughts go, the body follows – meaning that we have to harness the power of our thoughts and use willpower to protect ourselves from external forces that can ultimately bring us undone and manifest as disease.

We are faced with thousands of choices every day. Everything we do is a choice, from the moment we wake up until the moment we go to sleep. Health is a choice, inner peace is a choice, your life is a collection of the choices you have made. By choosing to establish strong mental and emotional boundaries, you may have to make some other new choices. If someone speaks to you about a problem, it only becomes your problem if you choose to take it on; until then you have complete control over your state of being. What you choose to consume, how you choose to live your life, the actions or movements you do or don't take, the reactions to your situations and your emotional responses are all a collection of choices that determine your quality of life. What do you want that to look like? The choice is yours.

To free your energy and create space for ultimate healing, work with your mind first, then your emotions and actions will have a strong foundation from which to blossom. Life is an adventure full of twists and turns, highs and lows, challenges and blessings – if we can begin to cultivate wisdom through our challenges, learn from our mistakes and foster compassion as we navigate the road to liberation, we will develop a deeper understanding of who we are and where our passions lie, and find the beauty in every situation – no matter how painful it can feel at the time. Look at your biggest challenges as your greatest teachers and believe that everything has a way of working itself out; everything is perfect just as it is.

AYURVEDIC
BEAUTY
ESSENTIALS

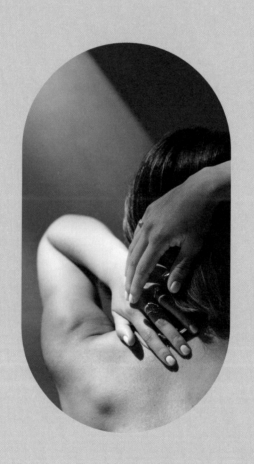

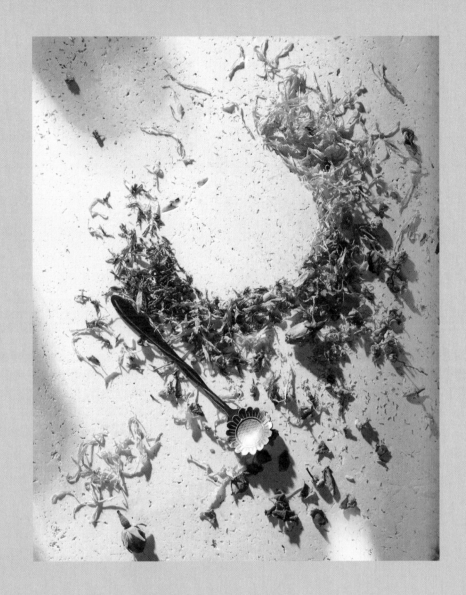

5

Understanding your skin

The appearance and characteristics of our skin are usually connected to our innate constitution, or Dosha. Each of the three Doshas has unique qualities that resemble its elemental makeup and reflect variations in the skin, which can help you to identify the best skincare regime for your personal, ever-changing needs.

Keep in mind that any imbalances you may be experiencing will need to be addressed first. For example, you may have Vata skin, which is naturally quite dry, but could be experiencing a Pitta imbalance, which would result in inflammation or acne, so Pitta would need to be pacified first. It's best to focus on how your skin is behaving at the moment (say, over the last month) and fine tune your regime if any changes occur.

Vata skin is dominated by the Air element, so by nature it has a tendency to be dry, thin, delicate and cold. Vata types are prone to wrinkles and premature ageing if ample oils are not included in both skincare and diet.

A Vata aggravation would look like dry, flaky skin that is thinning and sagging.

Vata skin is pacified by plenty of heavy oils, warming herbs and daily massage. It is best avoid excessive cleansing, exfoliating and abrasive scrubs as Vata skin needs a chance to develop its own natural oils.

Pitta skin is dominated by the Fire element, which makes it hot to the touch and moist/sweaty, and it can appear flushed. Pitta types have sensitive skin. They are the most likely to have freckles and moles, and can easily be sunburned.

A Pitta aggravation would include breakouts, acne, rosacea, inflammation, rashes, itchiness, a burning sensation, excessive oiliness and redness.

Pitta skin is pacified by light oils, cooling herbs, neem, absorbent flours and floral water.

Kapha skin is ruled by the Earth element, which makes it heavy, thick and rich with natural oils. Kapha skin is cool to touch, soft, smooth and supple, and remains plump.

A Kapha aggravation would manifest as enlarged, clogged pores, blackheads, excessive congestion and puffiness.

Kapha skin is pacified by minimal oils, warming herbs and facial steaming.

The characteristics of your skin will fluctuate as you float between the seasons, move between climates and navigate through life's experiences. Travel, air-conditioning and heating will also have an effect on your skin. Watch and observe, and use your wisdom to adjust your use of products as needed. The general rule is that dry skin needs heavy oils, moist skin needs light oils, rashes and inflammation need cooling herbs, and all skin needs time to breathe!

In terms of addressing specific skin conditions, Ayurveda seeks the root cause, which is rarely topical (unless you are experiencing a reaction to a current skincare product). The cause may be emotional, hormonal, lifestyle related or dietary, but until this cause is removed, skin conditions will remain. Focus on developing your daily routine, meditation and exercise practices, eating a wholesome diet, cleansing, utilising only natural skincare products and enjoying deep sleep for glowing skin.

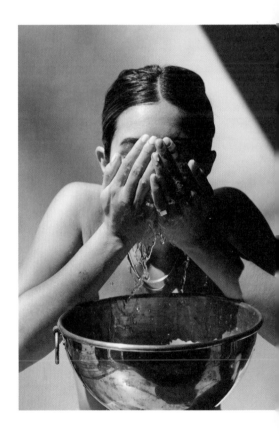

The fundamentals of beauty

Our physical appearance can be seen as a portal to our internal health. The state of our complexion, the strength of our nails and hair, and the lustre of our eyes are all gateways for understanding the inner workings of our body, mind and spirit.

When any of these quadrants are suffering, be it diet-related, emotional or due to a destructive lifestyle habit, messages will become visible in our physical appearance. This is our body's way of communicating with the conscious mind that an ailment lies within that needs to be addressed, giving us the opportunity to decipher exactly what the issue is so we can remedy the problem and regain our radiance. Paying attention to these signals puts you one step closer to becoming your own healer.

Beauty cannot be bought; there is no quick fix to glowing, radiant, ageless skin. Ayurveda lives by the adage that 'beauty comes from within'. As a holistic science, beauty is a result of living in alignment with nature, cultivating a wholesome diet, supporting digestive health and detoxification processes, achieving deep and rejuvenating sleep, honouring a complementary lifestyle, possessing a positive outlook and investing your time in self-care practices. When it comes to diet, whatever you put inside your body will express itself through the skin. By living within the sphere of Ayurvedic diet and lifestyle practices, you can expect to shine from the inside out.

As creatures of planet earth, we have been blessed by Mother Nature with all of the ingredients we need to live a happy and healthy life. Ayurveda honours the bounty of the plant kingdom and believes that everything we come into contact with should have natural roots. Our skin is the barrier between our internal habitat and the textures and energies of our environment; it is the connecting point between the innate and the external. As the skin is a major organ of absorption, it is vital to understand that everything we put on our skin will be absorbed directly into our bloodstream and carried into our liver for processing. Products containing chemicals and ingredients that are artificial pose a major threat to our entire system and their use can take years to manifest as health issues that are visible or diagnosable. As prevention is always a priority over cure, live by the notion that the products you use should be edible, so if you wouldn't eat it, don't put it on your skin.

The best way to ensure you are limiting your exposure to the harmful toxins found in modern beauty products is to opt to make your own at home using natural, organic and plant-based ingredients that nourish and hydrate your skin rather than strip and poison it. The art of crafting your own products is a beautiful tool for tapping in and connecting with the plant kingdom, developing an understanding of herbs, oils, flours and flowers and how they can imbue your life with soul. This is a perfect opportunity to draw upon the lineage of women from around the world who have utilised the healing powers of Mother Nature to nourish and nurture their skin since ancient times.

As a science that is so intrinsically intimate with nature, Ayurvedic beauty care is deeply rooted in plant-based products as well as the philosophy that less is more. Our skin needs to breathe – to gather Prana (life-force energy), connect with fresh oxygen and be given a chance to develop its own oils. By reducing your contact with multiple products, especially those which are quite dehydrating, and limiting abrasive scrubs and stripping soaps, your skin will be given the space to function as it was designed to.

Work within your environment. If you're living in a city and commuting to work, your skin will be exposed to pollution that needs to be cleansed. If you live within nature, or are on holidays in a luscious environment, your skin will require a lot less cleansing. As a basis, Ayurveda advocates minimal cleansing (which strips everything including your natural oils), nourishing your skin with nutrient-rich moisturising oils that nurture and protect, and massage to support lymphatic drainage, promote fresh blood supply, collagen production, muscle toning and detoxification.

Ayurveda has solutions for every ailment and provides natural, safe and nourishing alternatives for just about every store-bought personal care product. There is no need for a vanity cupboard full of products, these are items designed to be sold to you and they often contain very similar ingredients with alternative branding. Most of the recipes in this book have multiple uses so you can minimise the number of products on your shelf. All of the products are extremely cost-effective and can be made at home using simple ingredients from your kitchen pantry which you can trust are naturally derived, organic and totally edible. They also minimise your impact on the planet by reducing or eliminating the need for single-use plastics like toothpaste tubes and other plastic packaging that burden the environment. By opting to craft your own products, you can use glass and other reusable storage solutions that won't harm the planet.

Ageless beauty

Ageing is a rite of passage, a natural evolution as we journey through the human experience. With age comes knowledge, spiritual growth, maturity and exponential wisdom gained through overcoming life's challenges.

Each line, crease and crevice on a woman's body has been earned and should be worn with pride. In most Eastern cultures, older women are viewed as elders and are given great respect. When it comes to making important decisions, and for special guidance, their knowledge is sought after, as their years of experience have given them invaluable wisdom that simply can't be taught, only gained. Women are creators; we grow life, bear children, breastfeed and raise future generations. All of these gifts impact our physical appearance and it is only mainstream media that have told us these changes are not beautiful. But what could be more beautiful? We have been so conditioned to believe that youth equates to beauty and that being young and beautiful is synonymous with being a woman; we go out of our way and spend enormous amounts of money on products and procedures that claim to be anti-ageing, even when there are risks involved. Wouldn't it make more sense for us to reshape this mentality so that we are accepting and embracing of the natural phases of life and celebrate ageing as part of a the journey?

Our collagen production naturally begins to decline from around the age of twenty-five, which is when the signs of ageing begin to appear. It is tragic to think of a woman looking in the mirror for the rest of her life wishing she looked younger or hopelessly trying every avenue to regain youthful skin because of the outdated narrative we have been taught. The process of ageing is completely natural, it is inevitable and we have a responsibility to accept this as the truth and embrace the seasons of life with pride.

This isn't to say that taking care of your skin and investing in self-care practices is unnecessary. Quite the opposite. But the intention should be about embracing your natural foundations and indulging in the practices that nourish your soul and nurture your skin. Use these practices as an opportunity to step away from the superficiality and connect with yourself to develop a form of love and acceptance for the natural wonder that you are. The spiritual and emotional effect that self-love has on your physical appearance will far surpass any anti-ageing cream on the market.

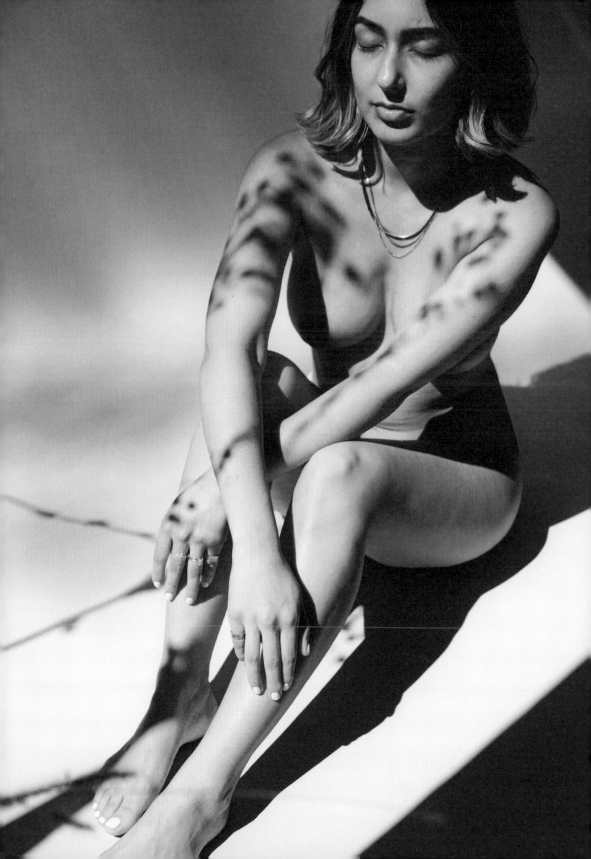

BEYOND THE PHYSICAL

There is no greater sense of beauty than that which comes from a person who loves the skin they're in, embraces their flaws, finds the perfection within the imperfection, and exudes kindness and compassion. Ayurveda dives deeper into the meaning of true beauty to include energetic attributes such as elegance, grace, kindness, softness, tenderness and optimism; as well as possessing good posture, graceful and conscious movement, a relaxed demeanour and a calm voice. Regardless of appearance, every individual has the opportunity to embody beauty by cultivating these innate qualities. Even the most typically attractive person can become unattractive through negative personality traits such as anger, jealousy, gossiping and selfishness. Embodying the qualities of a beautiful soul is one of the best-kept secrets in the treasure trove of Ayurvedic beauty gems.

Beauty lies in imperfection. Perfection is just a human construct designed to sell products. From day one we've been conditioned to believe that women should resemble what we see in magazines, advertisements and in Hollywood. Most of these images are so heavily edited that they themselves don't even represent women. We have a responsibility to undo this type of conditioning and learn to accept ourselves and others just as we are. What's more beautiful and empowering than a woman who is comfortable in her own skin?

How you visualise your own self-worth and self-image is also crucial to cultivating beauty. Everything your mind thinks, your body responds to, and this manifests as the energy you emit – some may call it your aura. If you look in the mirror and give your energy to the things you don't like, instead of the things you do, you are choosing to operate at a frequency that is not conducive to your highest self. Replace negative thoughts with positive, loving thoughts. Replace the limiting opinions you have about the things you don't like with the mantra that 'you are beautiful as you are'. This practice will rewire your neural pathways and you can begin to cultivate a more positive image of self-worth and self-love. Be compassionate, gentle and kind with yourself; speak to yourself only in the way that you would to your best friend.

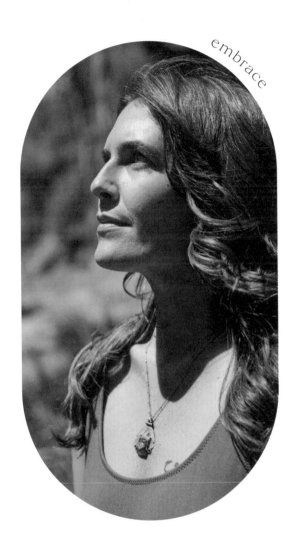

embrace

Crafting your own high-vibrational products

The treasure trove of plant-based ingredients Ayurveda promotes can often be found in your kitchen pantry; after all, they will be metabolised by your body just as food is, so they should be completely edible.

All of these ingredients have natural roots and contain the high-vibrational energy of plant magic. Plants are Mother Nature's gift to us. By utilising the knowledge of specific plants, you are working in alignment with the environment to protect your skin from the elements and to nourish your natural beauty throughout the seasons.

BEAUTY ESSENTIALS

Most of these ingredients are now available at supermarkets, organic grocery stores, health food stores, bulk food shops, local markets, online or from Asian/Indian supermarkets. Always opt for cold-pressed, raw, unrefined, organic brands where possible.

Oils

Make sure you opt for organic cold-pressed oils to ensure that the chemical compounds in the oil are not altered and there are no nasty additives.

o **Apricot kernel:** A lightweight oil known for its anti-ageing properties and suitability for most skin types due to its high content of vitamin E, which helps to calm inflamed skin. This is a great product for those new to using oil, as it won't block the pores and is easily absorbed.

o **Black sesame (untoasted):** Known as 'the king of oils', this is Ayurveda's most cherished of all oils and is nourishing for the entire body, from the tips of the toes to the scalp. Sesame oil easily penetrates the skin and is an excellent source of calcium, which helps to strengthen and support bone, muscle and joint health while protecting and moisturising the skin, hair and nails. Sesame oil has a unique fragrance that can take some getting used to; it can be disguised by blending other carrier oils or through the addition of essential oils. It is naturally warming, which helps to ground Vata and Kapha. Pitta types should use it sparingly, especially in summer. It is ideal for use on the body or blended with lighter oils for the face.

o **Castor:** When used topically, the cooling nature of castor oil helps to ease Pitta, calm skin irritations, balance skin flora and heal scalp issues. Castor oil has piercing properties that help to dissolve scar tissue and promote hair growth (it can be used across the eyelashes and brows). Castor oil has a viscous texture, so is best blended with other oils for a lighter finish.

o **Coconut:** Cooling in nature, this is the ideal oil for Pitta types or for use during summer when you are seeking a light layer of moisture that doesn't clog the pores. Coconut oil is soothing and hydrating and is packed full of nutrition to support healthy skin flora and protect it against the elements.

o **Ghee:** A very rich butter-based moisturiser that provides hydration to the deepest layers of the skin. The external use of ghee supports soft, supple skin by effectively helping to balance your skin's moisture levels and promote elasticity and skin rejuvenation.

o **Jojoba:** Perhaps the closest structure to the skin's natural sebum, jojoba agrees with almost every skin tone and type, making it the most versatile of all topical oils. Another great product to use when beginning your journey with oils.

o **Rosehip:** Ideal for mature skin, rosehip is thick and deeply nourishing for tired or aged skin that requires a more substantial amount of rejuvenation.

o **Sweet almond:** A very light oil that is packed full of nutrients to smooth, soften and heal skin ailments by stimulating the production of new skin cells, smoothing fine lines and healing skin damage. Suitable for all skin types.

Plants

o **Calendula:** An incredibly soothing plant that has long been used for its abilities to restore skin, assist in wound healing and activate collagen production while offering protection from skin ailments and external damage. Known to heal inflammation, psoriasis, rashes, age spots, dermatitis, varicose veins, stretch marks and warts.

o **Chamomile:** Another soothing plant, it is known for its ability to heal skin irritations, burns and acne while diminishing the development of wrinkles.

o **Hibiscus:** Rich in vitamin C, hibiscus is renowned for prolonging the longevity of the skin and improving the complexion and elasticity while reducing age spots and acne, and detoxifying the skin. A must-have in your skincare regime.

o **Lavender:** With an ability to calm and soothe many conditions, lavender is especially beneficial in reducing inflammation, acne and premature ageing while eliminating unwanted bacteria from the skin.

o **Neem:** The extremely bitter nature and sulphur content of the neem plant give it its anti-inflammatory wound-healing abilities, which help to soothe and heal all skin ailments, from insect bites to infections. It is also effective in combating acne and premature ageing, reducing rashes, eliminating unwanted bacteria and even preventing greying. Another must-have ingredient.

o **Nettles:** Rich in vitamins, nutrients and sulphur, nettles boost collagen receptors that keep skin youthful. They are often used in beauty products for their restorative and reparative properties.

o **Rose:** Cooling and soothing by nature, rose is effective in reducing Pitta conditions such as inflammation, acne, rosacea, eczema and rashes while providing moisture and hydration to the skin. Packed with vitamins, rose helps to prevent premature ageing, smooth fine lines, reduce the look of age spots and aid with collagen production.

o **Sage:** Rich in antioxidants, astringent properties and antibacterial qualities, sage leaves are ideal for oily, wrinkled or saggy skin. These leaves will primarily clean and restore elasticity to your skin.

o **Triphala:** A cherished Ayurvedic formula composed of the powders of three dried fruits: amalaki, bibhitaki and haritaki; Triphala is revered for its unique ability to gently cleanse and detoxify the entire body, and when used topically provides deep cleansing, rebalancing and nutritive qualities that work to harmonise all Doshas. Triphala is extremely versatile and can be used as a body cleanser, toothpaste, hair mask, eyewash etc. Triphala is a must-have for anyone beginning their Ayurvedic journey.

o **Tulsi:** Known as 'holy basil', Tulsi has antifungal and antibiotic properties that work to boost skin tone, clear blemishes and rejuvenate the skin.

o **Turmeric:** The antiseptic and anti-inflammatory properties of turmeric help to soothe all skin ailments, while the antioxidants and nutritive value defend and protect the skin for a youthful appearance.

Flours

o **Arrowroot and cornstarch:** Both of these flours are used to absorb excess liquid, which is beneficial in products like deodorant and dry shampoo, where the intention is to reduce moisture.

o **Besan/chickpea:** A very versatile, nutrient-dense flour with the ability to reduce skin oiliness, acne, inflammation, clogged pores and facial hair, and gently exfoliate dead skin cells, promoting fresh, youthful, glowing skin.

Clays

All clays are essentially forms of soil that are rich in vitamins and minerals with amazing cleansing and purifying properties for the skin. When applied, clay draws out oil and impurities, refines pores and detoxifies the skin, leaving it balanced and clean. As they are absorbent by nature, it is important to find a suitable clay for your skin type, otherwise they can be dehydrating.

o **Bentonite:** A silky clay created from volcanic ash with highly absorbent qualities. Ideal for oily or congested skin. Suitable for Kapha skin types who are aged twenty-five and over.

o **Green:** A soft, green granular clay created from decomposed plant matter and iron oxides. It's best suited to oily, inflamed and irritated Pitta skin types. Suitable for youths.

o **Pink:** A light, rose-tinted clay suitable for sensitive, dry and mature skin due to its gentle nature. Suitable for Vata skin types.

Other

o **Aloe vera gel:** Naturally cooling, aloe vera gel is highly soothing for irritated, inflamed or sensitive skin. The antibacterial nature of this plump gel makes it an ideal base for face and body cleansers and improves oral hygiene. Ideal for Pitta types or in cases of burns, dryness or for the relief of skin disorders.

o **Beeswax:** A natural by-product from the production of honey, beeswax provides deep nutrition for dry or irritated skin while providing a stable base for hearty personal care products such as body butter and lip balm.

o **Bicarbonate of soda (baking soda):** A natural mineral sourced from soda ash from evaporated lake basins, it has a vast array of purposes, from household cleaners through to personal care products like toothpaste, deodorant and shampoo etc. The antibacterial nature of bicarbonate of soda (baking soda) assists with skin irritations and detoxification, while the granular texture makes it mildly exfoliating.

o **Castille soap:** A foamy, natural liquid soap derived from plant-based vegetable oils that contains no nasty additives or chemicals. Perfect for the face, body and hair. A nice addition to homemade cleansers due to its foamy consistency.

o **Candelilla wax:** A lightweight wax derived from a small shrub that provides a plant-based alternative to beeswax and is especially popular in lip balms due to its glossy finish.

o **Honey:** Packed full of antibacterial, anti-inflammatory, antiseptic and antibiotic properties, honey has been used for thousands of years to treat skin conditions by rebalancing flora, purifying the skin and providing relief from irritations and dryness.

o **Lemon:** The high levels of vitamin C found in lemons help to detoxify, cleanse the pores and brighten the complexion while removing dead skin and excess oil.

o **Shea butter:** A plant-based fat derived from the shea nut, shea butter provides deep nutrition and hydration to dry skin while soothing inflammation. This is the heaviest of all skin salves, so it should be used sparingly by Pitta types or in the summer. Ideal for dry, mature Vata skin.

o **Essential oils:** For a complete guide to the aromatic and healing powers of essential oils refer to *A Scented Life* by Pat Princi-Jones.

BOTANICAL OIL BLENDS

There is an entire ecosystem of essential bacteria living on the surface of your face and body that protects and promotes the longevity of your skin. This bacteria will naturally defend you from toxins and pollution, so the goal is not to strip them away, but rather feed them with healthy nutrients to support their form and function, and that's exactly what plant-based oils do. Most store-bought beauty products are filled with chemicals that destroy this perfect balance, so it's best to opt for oils infused with the healing powers of the plant kingdom for healthy, glowing skin.

Beginning your journey with oils can be intimidating at first if you have never used them before. A lot of people assume they will clog the pores and cause bumps or irritation. I can assure you there is an oil for everyone; it's just about experimenting and finding the one that works for your skin type. Start out by trying one of the lighter recommended oils straight for one week and see how your skin responds to it. Pick the one that calls out to you the most. You can even smell each and allow your senses to guide you. Fragrances with the most appealing aroma can indicate what the body is craving and will be the most compatible. Once you find your soul match, you will never look back. Not only are oils 100 per cent natural, they are beneficial to the whole body (inside and out) while adding the most luscious glow to the skin; they are also incredibly cost effective and zero-waste when bought in bulk.

Dried flowers and plants infuse oils with even more power. Experiment with the plants that resonate with you and your needs. I like to keep a 1 litre jar of black sesame oil full of my favourite dried flowers sitting on my kitchen windowsill, as the sun infuses its healing powers into the oil. I'll use this as my base oil for all of my products throughout the month.

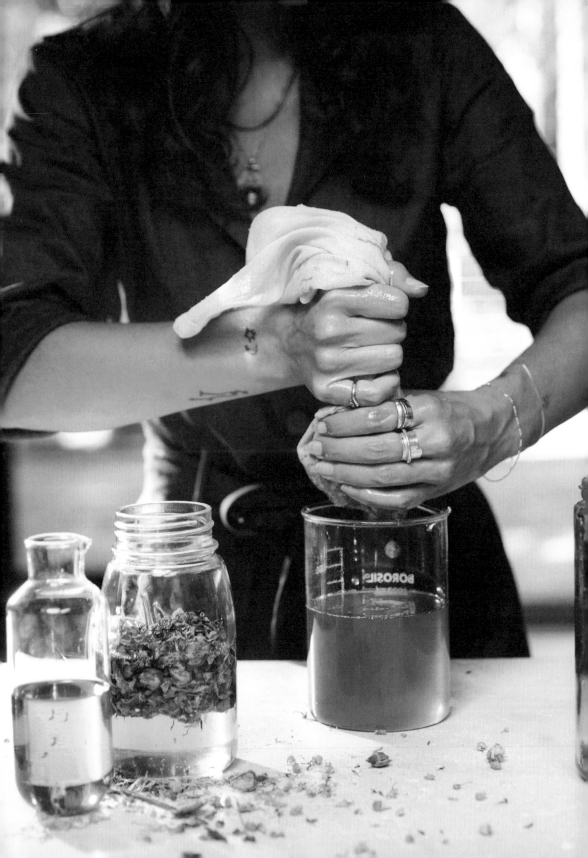

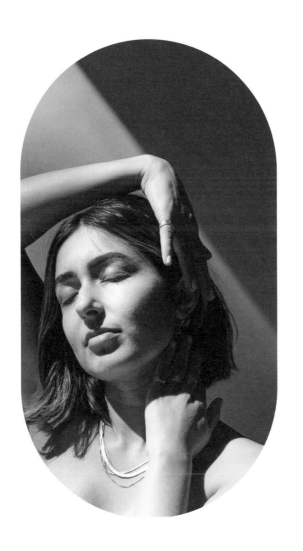

Floral base oil

This luscious infusion provides a plant-adorned oil which can be used as the basis for all of your personal care products.

Makes 250 ml (8½ fl oz)

250 ml (8½ fl oz) raw black sesame oil (untoasted)

250 g (9 oz) dried flowers of your choice (see page 72)

Add the dried flowers to a 500 ml (17 fl oz) sterilised glass jar. Ensure there is absolutely no water in the jar before beginning, as this will breed mould.

Top the jar with oil, pop the lid on and roll the jar on its side a few times to mix everything together. Then choose one of the infusion methods listed below.

Solar infusion: Sit the jar in a sunny spot for up to 3 weeks, turning the jar once a day.

Heat infusion: Cook over very low heat (around 30°C [70°F]) so you don't spoil the medicinal properties of the plants) for 3 hours.

Strain the plant matter out completely using a nut milk bag.

TIP: Fresh plants can be used but must be completely dry and strained thoroughly, as they can become mouldy and the water content can spoil oils.

Body/Abhyanga oil

The body benefits largely both from the nutritive qualities of herbal oil and the physical benefits of massage and touch – see page 56 to learn more about the practice of Abhyanga.

Makes 500 ml (17 fl oz)

250 ml (8 ½ fl oz) floral base oil (see page 78)

250 ml (8 ½ fl oz) carrier oil suited to your Dosha (see page 72)

Combine all of the ingredients in a sterilised glass jar.

Put the lid on, swirl to blend and store out of direct sunlight.

Face oil

This oil is packed with vitamins, minerals and antioxidants perfectly suited to your face. Simply use this as a base and finish with some lighter oils and essential oils based on your needs.

Makes 100 ml (3½ fl oz)

50 ml (1¾ fl oz) floral base oil (see page 78)

2 tablespoons face oil of your choice (see below for recommendations)

2 teaspoons castor oil

10 drops of essential oil (frankincense, myrrh, rose, geranium, chamomile, lavender etc.)

Add 50 ml (1¾ fl oz) of the floral base oil to a 100 ml (3½ fl oz) sterilised glass jar.

Add face oil of your choice.

Add the castor oil.

Put the lid on, swirl a few times and store out of direct sunlight.

TIP: If you are new to using oil on your skin and have small pores or reactive/sensitive skin, you may like to begin with apricot kernel oil, as it is very light and will not clog the pores, or jojoba, which is the closest to the skin's natural sebum (oils).

Tridoshic face oil blend

This is a simple recipe with suggested face and essential oils that suit all skin types. A great place to start your relationship with face oils.

Makes 100 ml (3½ fl oz)

50 ml (1¾ fl oz) floral base oil (see page 78) or plain black sesame oil

1 tablespoon sweet almond oil

1 tablespoon apricot kernel oil

2 teaspoons castor oil

10 drops of rose geranium essential oil

5 drops of lavender essential oil

Combine all ingredients in a sterilised glass jar.

Put the lid on, swirl to blend and store out of direct sunlight.

Tridoshic moisturising face + body cleanser

Our skincare regime begins with our cleanser. The goal is not to strip the skin, but to support the millions of microbiomes (good bacteria) that live on the skin and work to protect and keep the skin barrier functioning. When the microbiome is not in equilibrium (due to harsh chemicals, soaps, exfoliants, sulphates, hair removal products, makeup etc.), we begin to see skin conditions flaring up. Less is more! The closer your products are to your skin's sebum (natural oils) and pH level, the less likely they are to interfere with the balance of bacteria that allow your skin to remain plump, healthy and glowing.

Makes 50 ml (1¾ fl oz)

3 tablespoons aloe vera gel

1 teaspoon fractionated coconut oil (optional)

5 drops of lavender essential oil

5 drops of rose geranium essential oil

3 tablespoons rosewater

1 tablespoon lemon juice

1 teaspoon raw honey

1 teaspoon Triphala powder

¼ teaspoon sea salt

25 ml (¾ fl oz) or 100 ml (3½ fl oz) castile soap (optional, see tip below)

Add the aloe vera gel, coconut oil, if using, and essential oils to a glass jar and mix well. Allow this mix to sit for 10 minutes to emulsify/bind the ingredients together.

Add the remaining ingredients and stir to combine.

Store in a squeeze tube for easy access or a glass jar.

Try to keep this product away from running water and excess heat to extend its shelf life.

If making a body wash or foaming face wash, add 50 ml of castile soap.

TIP: Aloe vera gel creates the gel-like consistency that forms the base. All of the remaining ingredients can be optional, so if you prefer not to use any of them, or have trouble finding them, simply omit them from the ingredients.

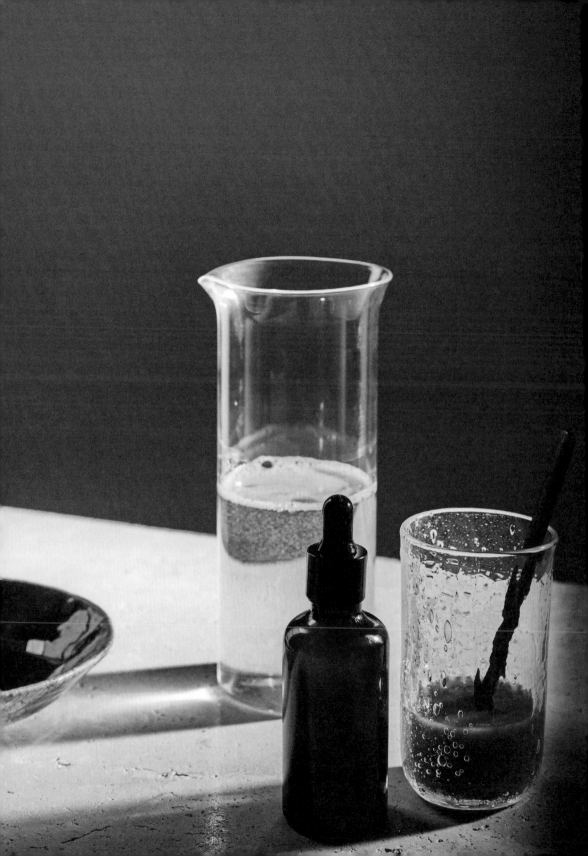

Tridoshic gentle exfoliant 'Ubtan'

Exfoliants are often too abrasive for the gentle nature of the skin on our face but 'Ubtans' have been used for thousands of years to remove dead skin cells, wash away impurities and dissolve any build-up of products we may have accumulated. They are gentle enough for daily or weekly use and can also be applied as a mask. Crafted with raw, nutritive grains and herbal powders, they cleanse, improve circulation and strengthen the skin.

Makes 300 ml (10 fl oz)

1 cup (120 g 4 ½ oz) besan (chickpea flour)

2 tablespoons clay (see below for suitable clay for your skin type)

1 tablespoon Triphala powder

1 teaspoon neem powder (optional)

2 teaspoons hibiscus or rose powder (optional)

Clay for your skin type:

VATA (dry/mature):
pink or red clay

PITTA (red/oily/inflamed):
green clay

KAPHA (oily/congested):
pink or bentonite clay

Mix all of the ingredients in a small bowl.

Store them in a glass jar with it's lid on.

How to apply:

As a scrub: Wet your face with warm water, take 1 teaspoon of the Ubtan mix and massage it into your skin. Remove with a damp facecloth or wet hands.

As a mask: Put 1 teaspoon of the Ubtan mix in a small bowl or cup and slowly stir in a few drops of water to make a moist paste.

Wash your face and apply the mask in upward strokes, beginning with your chin.

Allow the mask to set, then leave it on for 2–10 minutes, removing it with downward motions using a damp facecloth or wet hands. You want to remove the mask before it's overly dry and abrasive.

TIP: You can use the besan on its own; all of the other ingredients are optional and interchangeable.

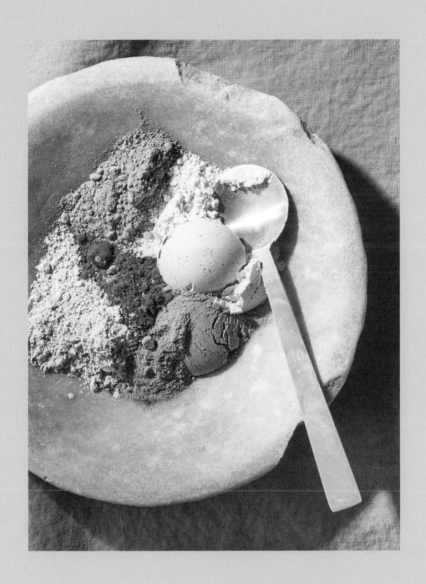

Nourishing lip balm

Anything we apply to the lips will certainly make its way into the mouth, so it's crucial these products are completely natural and edible! Candelilla is a plant-based wax often used for lip balms, as it has a glossy finish. If you prefer a more neutral look, opt for soy wax, which is vegan, or beeswax, derived from honey.

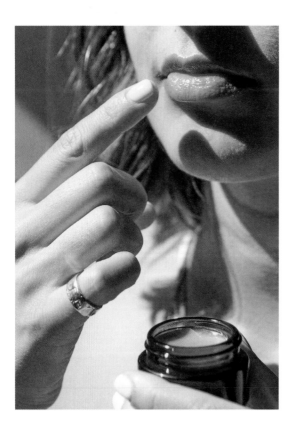

Makes 50 ml (1 ¾ fl oz)

1 teaspoon candelilla wax

2 teaspoons shea butter

4 teaspoons coconut oil

2 teaspoons castor oil

Melt the candelilla wax in a metal mixing bowl over a small pot of boiling water until the wax is completely liquid.

Add the shea butter and coconut oil, melting until liquid.

Remove from the heat and add the castor oil.

Stir to combine, then pour into a small glass jar for use with a lid and allow it to set in the fridge for around 30 minutes.

TIP: Avoid using essential oils on anything that goes near the mouth, as the taste can be overpowering.

You can create tints by adding ground beetroot, hibiscus, cacao, cinnamon, turmeric etc. to the mixture when you add the oils. Experiment with colours of your choice. This works as a cheek tint also.

Rejuvenating eye cream

The skin around the eyes is the most delicate of the whole body and is prone to lose strength and elasticity. This rejuvenating eye cream feeds the deepest layers of the skin, providing healthy fats that protect and promote longevity. This is a very simple recipe that uses only three ingredients, which have all been used for thousands of years to support vision and soothe the eyes, while promoting the growth of eyelashes and eyebrows.

Makes 50 ml (1 ¾ fl oz)

1 tablespoon ghee, melted

1 tablespoon coconut oil, melted

10 ml castor oil

Melt the ghee and coconut oil in a metal mixing bowl over a small pot of boiling water until completely liquid.

Remove from the heat and add the castor oil.

Stir to combine, then pour into a small sterilised glass jar, with a lid, for use.

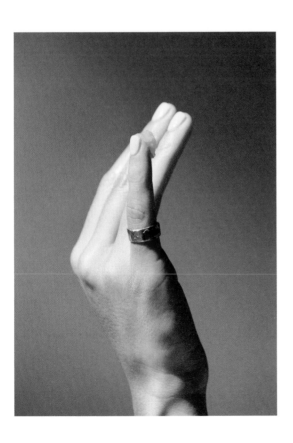

TIP: Before bed each night, apply this cream liberally across the whole eye, under the eyes and across the eyelashes and eyebrows.

This is a wonderful all-round beauty butter that can also be used as a lip balm, hand cream, salve, and is very nourishing for dry skin particularly around the elbows and heels.

Luscious rose body butter

A wonderful all-over body butter that is deeply moisturising and protective. It can be used to provide nourishment to the skin, hands, nails, cuticles, feet, heels, elbows and knees; to support the skin during pregnancy and prevent stretch marks; or as a soothing baby cream. This cream is also very effective in healing and reducing scar tissue or can be massaged into various parts of the body that may benefit from some extra TLC, such as the heart, breasts or externally over the womb.

Makes 285 g (10 oz)

200ml shea butter, melted

1 tablespoon coconut oil

1 tablespoon castor oil

½ cup (125 ml/4 fl oz) jojoba, sweet almond or floral base oil (see page 78)

1–2 teaspoons dried rose powder

10–15 drops of rose essential oil (optional)

Heat 5 cm (2 in) of water in a large saucepan on the lowest heat to create a double boiler. Add the shea butter and coconut oil to a glass beaker or heat-proof glass jar and place it in the water until the oils have completely melted (about 20 minutes).

Remove the beaker from the heat and place it in the freezer for about 45 minutes until it begins to firm up but is still soft enough to whip.

Pour the mixture into a large mixing bowl and add the remaining ingredients, using between 1–2 teaspoons of rose powder depending how pink you would like it to be. Use a handheld or electric whisk to create a luscious, creamy butter much like whipped cream.

Scoop into a sterilised glass jar, with a lid and allow it to set in the fridge for 30 minutes.

TIP: Avoid using essential oils for baby cream or natural sex lubricant.

This makes a wonderful gift; top with a few dried rose petals in a nice glass jar.

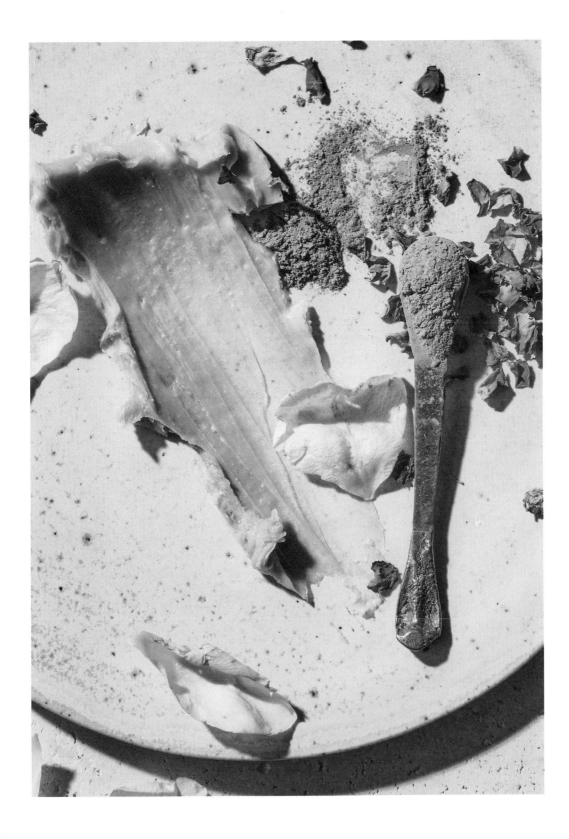

Rehydrating hair treatment

It's common for hair to dry out due to changes in season, exposure to the sun, salt or chlorinated water, hair dye, styling tools and toxic hair products, which can all cause the hair to break, frizz and thin out, and result in issues such as dandruff, loss of growth and discolouration. Using a few edible ingredients, you can nourish the scalp, strengthen the hair and protect it from the elements, giving you more luscious, vibrant locks.

Makes 1 mask for shoulder-length hair

2 tablespoons besan (chickpea flour)

¼ teaspoon Triphala powder or ground cinnamon

¼ teaspoon neem powder (prevents greying and relieves dandruff)

1 teaspoon black sesame oil or floral base oil (see page 78)

1 teaspoon castor oil

½ cup (125 g/4½ oz) coconut yoghurt

10 drops of lavender essential oil (soothes the scalp)

Mix the dry ingredients in a bowl and slowly stir in the wet ingredient.

How to apply:

Apply to clean, damp hair with your fingertips, starting at the scalp and working your way down to the ends.

Once evenly applied, gently massage for 1–3 minutes and then wrap your hair in a bun and cover with a shower cap for up to 20 minutes.

Rinse out with lukewarm water and a gentle natural shampoo.

TIP: You can double or halve the recipe, depending on the length of your hair.

Volumising dry shampoo

Using dry shampoo is an effective way to reduce the frequency of washing your hair, which can strip the essential natural oils needed to protect the hair and keep the scalp hydrated and healthy. This recipe provides extra nutrition, improving the strength of your hair while adding volume and body. The colour can be adapted to suit your base colour by adding a few medicinal spices.

Makes 50 g (1 ¾ oz)

3 tablespoons arrowroot flour or cornstarch

Optional:

1 teaspoon lavender powder (soothes dandruff & dry scalp, imbues floral aroma)

1 teaspoon sage powder (promotes hair growth & prevents greying)

1 teaspoon aloe vera powder (hydrating for dry scalp and brittle hair)

2 teaspoons hair tint to suit your hair tone (see variations below)

Red, blonde or sandy hair: Cinnamon, turmeric, cacao & red clay.

Brown or black hair: Cacao, charcoal & green clay.

Blend the tint to suit your hair tone in a small bowl.

Add remaining ingredients, mix and store in a glass jar.

How to apply:

Tie your hair back (unless your hair is very short) and use a blush brush to apply the mix across your hairline.

Take your hair out and apply more powder along your part line.

Massage the powder into the roots and brush through to finish.

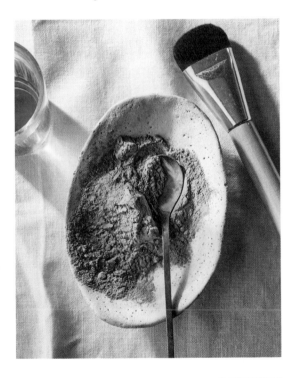

TIP: This product can also be used as a powdered face foundation to absorb excess oil and provide some coverage.

Neutralising deodorant

Under our arms lives a portal to our lymphatic system, so it's vital that all products used in this area are completely natural. The rate at which we perspire is largely based on our diet, so by adopting an Ayurvedic diet you should find that this area becomes a lot more discreet. This recipe has qualities that are both absorbent and odour neutralising while supporting healthy detoxification.

Makes 100 g (3 ½ oz)

2 tablespoons shea butter

1 teaspoon coconut oil

3 tablespoons cornstarch or arrowroot powder (for absorbancy)

½ teaspoon bicarbonate soda

15–20 drops of essential oils of your choice

Melt the shea butter and coconut oil in a metal mixing bowl over a small pot of boiling water until completely liquid.

Remove from the heat and add the cornstarch or arrowroot powder and bicarbonate of soda.

Mix well to ensure no lumps are left behind.

Add the essential oils, stir to combine.

Pour into a small sterilised glass jar, with a lid, for use.

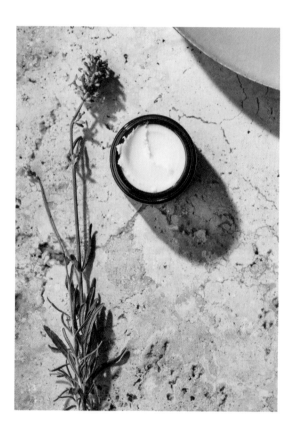

TIP: For a floral aroma, try 10 drops of rose, 5 drops of lavender and 5 drops of ylang ylang oil.

For an earthy aroma, try 10 drops of patchouli, 5 drops of bergamot and 5 drops of cedar or sandalwood oil.

Natural fragrances, body mists and toners

Floral waters make an amazing and totally natural base for crafting perfumes, natural deodorants and refreshing fragrant mists that add moisture to the skin before applying oils or creams, as well as rehydrating the skin throughout the day.

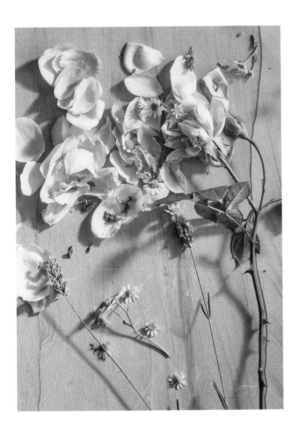

Makes 100 ml (3½ fl oz)

Base: 80 ml (2½ fl oz) base water – choose from the following:

rosewater

orange blossom water

chamomile tea (supports relaxation and sleep)

sage tea (for oily skin)

neem tea (for skin irritations or acne)

1 teaspoon fractionated coconut oil (optional)

1 teaspoon aloe vera gel (cooling, perfect for after-sun use)

essential oils of your choice

Pour all of the ingredients you have chosen to use into a 100 ml (3½ fl oz) spray jar, secure the spray lid and shake to combine.

> **TIP:** You may like to use the floral water on its own if using on the face. For fragrances, use up to 20 drops of your favourite essential oils based on how strong you would like the aroma.

Refreshing floral mouthwash

Mouthwash should cleanse the palate and refresh the breath, remove debris and moisturise the gums, not strip healthy bacteria that live within the mouth and are needed for oral health. This gentle mouthwash won't disrupt your natural balance, as it supports gum and tooth health. Aloe vera accelerates healing and is effective in treating cavities, as it inhibits the growth of the bacteria that causes dental decay.

Makes 250 ml (8½ fl oz)

150 ml (5 fl oz) aloe vera juice

100 ml (3 ½ fl oz) rosewater

½ teaspoon stevia

10 drops of peppermint oil

5 drops of spearmint oil

5 drops of fennel oil

Combine all of the ingredients in a sterilised glass jar.

Put the lid on and swirl to blend.

Swirl before each use.

Antibacterial toothpaste

Nature provides all of the ingredients we need to support oral hygiene. This recipe is easy to make and packed full of antibacterial ingredients, and you can craft a flavour based on essential oils of your choice.

Makes 200 ml (7 fl oz)

¼ cup (55 g/2 oz) coconut oil

½ cup (120 g/4½ oz) bicarbonate of soda

1 teaspoon Triphala (herbal preparation)

1 teaspoon stevia (plant-based sweetener, optional)

1 teaspoon bentonite or green clay (optional)

10–15 drops of essential oils such as peppermint, fennel, lemon, sage, rosemary, clove, cinnamon or orange

5 drops of neem seed oil (optional)

Melt the coconut oil in a small saucepan.

Remove it from the heat and slowly mix in the bicarbonate of soda.

Add in the remaining ingredients, stir well, pour into a sterilised glass jar, with a lid and allow to set in the fridge for 15 minutes.

TIP: remove the Triphala and clay for a colourless version.

Oil pulling blend

Makes 100 ml (3½ fl oz)

*40 ml (⅓ fl oz) (untoasted, raw)
black sesame oil*

*60 ml (2 fl oz) fractionated coconut oil
(liquid coconut oil)*

*10 drops of essential oils: sage, fennel,
mint, cinnamon, clove etc. (optional)*

Combine all of the ingredients in
a sterilised glass jar. Put the lid on
and swirl to blend.

Swirl before each use.

Place approximately 2–3 teaspoons
of oil in the mouth and gently swish
back and forth, occasionally pulling
the oil through the teeth.

Continue this practice for anywhere
between 1 minute and 20 minutes
(the longer - the better the results).
You may like to do this while you're
showering.

Spit the oil out and rinse with warm
water or a gentle mouthwash.

*TIP: Oil can clog the drain so it's
recommended to spit it out in
the garden or bin.*

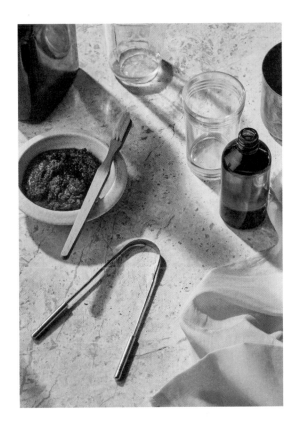

SELF-CARE RITUALS

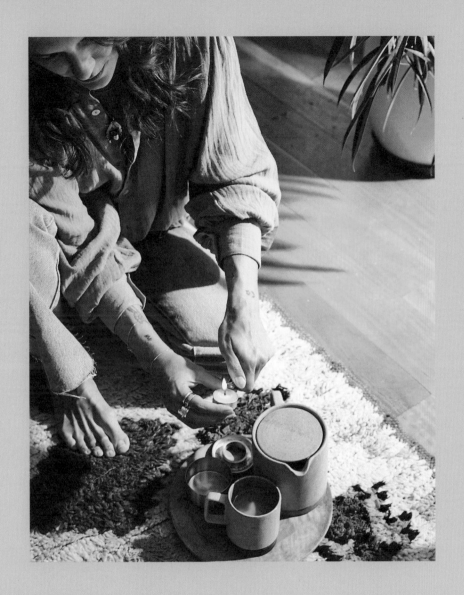

Ayurveda offers many beautiful self-care practices that you can follow from the comfort of your own home, using simple ingredients and tools. These practices are designed to help you slow down and nourish yourself. They are particularly potent during times of heightened emotion, stress and insomnia as they allow your body to become flooded with a sense of inner peace. Have fun exploring the various techniques and don't be afraid to adapt them to suit your own personal style.

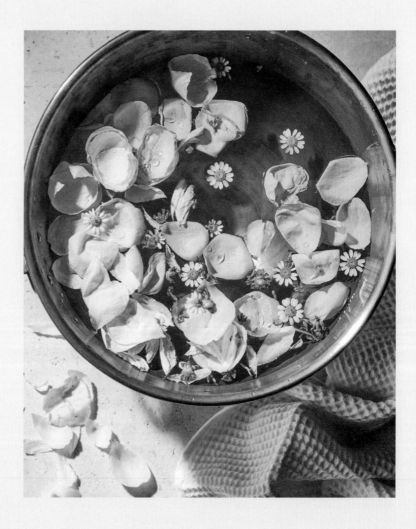

Face steaming (Swedana)

This beautiful, sensorial experience is warming, grounding, detoxifying and therapeutic, alleviating congestion and allergies. It also prepares your skin for other treatments. Facial steaming also sharpens mental clarity and improves sleep.

3 cups (750 ml/25½ fl oz) filtered water

2 drops of essential oil/s of your choice (lemon myrtle, eucalyptus, lavender, chamomile, rosemary etc.)

1 tablespoon rosewater (optional)

1 teaspoon fresh or dried calendula, lavender, rose petals, hibiscus and/or chrysanthemum

Either add all of the ingredients to a bowl and top with boiling water or simmer all of the dried ingredients and water in a pot, covered, for 10 minutes; add the rosewater and essential oils once removed from the heat. If boiled in a pot, transfer to a large bowl.

Lean over the bowl and place a towel over your head so the steam can't escape, with a gap of 10-15 cm (4-6 in) between your face and the hot water.

With your eyes closed, meditate and breathe deeply through your nose for 5-10 minutes.

Gently pat your face dry with a towel, spritz your skin with a floral toner and apply facial oil in an upwards motion.

Face massage

Below the surface of our supple skin lives lymphatic fluid that helps to drain and detoxify the skin's impurities. Massage also helps with detoxification while sending fresh blood to the skin's surface, which restores skin cells and improves collagen production, as well as keeping the muscles of the face toned.

After cleansing, apply a floral water toner and a generous amount of face oil.

Begin massaging in long strokes from the base of the neck up to the chin to open up the channels for lymphatic drainage.

Using your thumbs and index fingers, glide along the jawline from the chin to the ear.

Repeat this process along the cheekbone.

Massage the gland found next to each nostril, at the bridge of the nose under the eye, at the hairline end of the cheekbone, and just underneath where your inner eyebrow begins.

Pinch your fingers along the eyebrow, heading towards the hairline.

Use your fingertips to massage the forehead from the midline to the hairline.

Repeat this entire process in reverse to coax the lymphatic fluid out of the face, ending in downward strokes on the neck.

The Ayurvedic facial

Ayurveda provides a truly decadent ritual that will leave you nourished and glowing both on the inside and outside. You may like to do this if you're experiencing some inflammation, a breakout, dryness, or just feel like indulging. For a quick version you can skip the massage and steam; simply cleanse and apply the mask!

1 tablespoon flour (oat or chickpea)

⅛ teaspoon turmeric powder

¼ teaspoon coriander (cilantro) powder

½ teaspoon Triphala powder

1 teaspoon rosewater or milk of your choice

For Vata (dry, dehydrated or mature skin), add:

1 teaspoon red clay

¼ teaspoon rose powder (optional)

1 teaspoon sesame oil or castor oil

For Pitta (red, itchy or blemished skin), add:

1 teaspoon green clay

¼ teaspoon neem powder

¼ teaspoon lavender powder (optional)

1 teaspoon coconut or sweet almond oil

For Kapha (oily, congested skin), add:

1 teaspoon red or bentonite clay

1 teaspoon ground orange peel (optional)

¼ teaspoon rose powder (optional)

1 teaspoon sesame oil

Begin by cleansing the skin. Indulge in a facial massage targeting specific points to release tension, followed by a facial steam (see page 97).

Mix the flour and ground herbs together in a small mixing bowl, using your hands or a spoon.

Stir the oil in slowly to blend.

Slowly add water or milk to reach the desired consistency. The paste should be moist enough to apply but firm enough to dry on the skin.

Apply the paste in upward motions, beginning along the jawline towards the hairline. You may like to include your neck and décolletage also.

Lie back and enjoy the relaxing and intoxicating qualities of the aromas.

After 5-10 minutes, moisten a washcloth with warm water and begin to remove the mask in downward motions, beginning from the hairline.

Once the mask is removed, spray your face with some rosewater to tone, and massage a light face oil into the skin in upwards motions.

TIP: For a quick version you can skip the massage and steam; simply cleanse and apply mask!

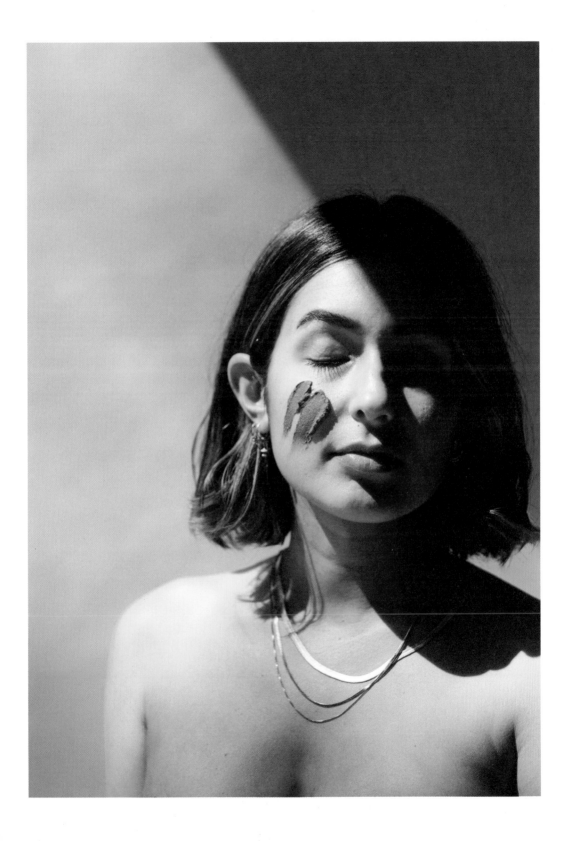

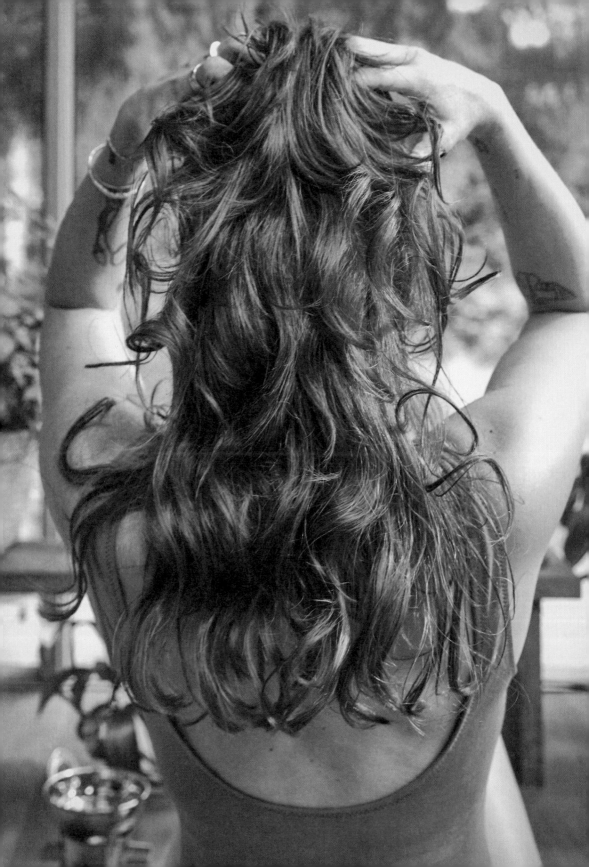

Head/scalp massage (Shiro Abhyanga)

The home of our five senses lies within our head. We receive a lot of experiences through this direct portal, so it's important to nourish and keep the conscious connection alive. Head massage is the most intimate therapy we can do for mental stimulation and cognitive function, which largely affects our sleep, vision, energy, emotions, memory and all of our motor skills. This practice also helps to calm the nervous system and balance hormones. Massaging our scalp also helps to stimulate hair growth and improve the strength and length of hair. A wonderful practice before bedtime for a relaxing night's sleep.

Warm a blend of 2 tablespoons black sesame and 1 teaspoon castor oil; set this aside in a small dish. Add a few drops of neem oil to relieve dandruff, hair loss or greying.

Rub some oil onto the fingertips and, pulsing the fingers, glide them from your hairline to the crown of your head to spread the oil. You don't want to drag your fingers over the hair; this is about targeting the scalp itself.

Once the scalp is moist with oil, massage your entire head in small, circular motions with the tips of the fingers, using firm pressure. Always work up to the crown.

Focus some attention on the temples, the crown of the head and the two points where the skull meets the top of the neck.

Finish by pressing the palms together on either side of the skull in clockwise motions.

For best results, leave the oil in for 20 minutes, or overnight.

Foot massage

As the far extremities of the body – and the connective point between ourselves and the earth – the feet hold a lot of tension. By working to relax them, you are inviting the whole body to ground down into earth energy. Our feet are largely connected to our eyes, so this practice also helps to rejuvenate our senses. This is one of the best therapies for curing insomnia. Pop some oil on your bedside table and spend 10 minutes massaging your feet for a deep night's sleep.

Warm 2 tablespoons black sesame oil with grounding essential oils of your choice (cedarwood, geranium, patchouli, sandalwood, lavender etc.); set aside in a dish.

Find a comfortable position and cradle your right foot. Apply some warm oil all over the foot.

Glide your thumbs up the arch of your foot, paying particular attention to the midline, outer edges and the ball of the foot.

Use your flat palm to draw a figure of 8 motion across the sole.

Squeeze your foot with both hands along the outer edges, up and down the foot.

Massage each toe from the base to the tip and include the space between the toes.

Hold your toes and rotate the foot in both directions. Point and flex the foot a few times.

Turn your foot over and glide your thumbs up and down the grooves between the bones on the top of your foot.

Massage each toe using circular motions over the joints. Massage the nail and nail bed.

Pull your toes up towards your shin then curl them over.

Finish by massaging the back of the heel up to the base of the calf with long strokes, and use clockwise motions around the ankle.

Repeat with your left foot.

Foot bath

Bathing your feet in warm water with a lovely blend of salts and flowers is a very grounding and effective tool for unwinding after a long day, especially if you've been running around in uncomfortable shoes. The use of salts helps to draw out any impurities and is very detoxifying. This is a wonderful practice to prepare for a foot massage, by cleansing and softening the tissues, or to do after a foot massage, to cleanse away any toxins that have been released.

Prepare a foot bath or a large bucket with warm to hot water. Add 1 cup dried flowers of your choice and 5–10 drops of essential oils; you can add ½ cup epsom salts for inflammation/swelling, 1 teaspoon ground ginger if you have poor circulation, or fennel seeds and mint leaves for a cooling effect.

Submerge your feet in the water for 10–15 minutes, or as long as the water stays warm. Relax, breathe deeply and sink into this luxurious sensation as you unwind.

Pat your feet dry with a towel and apply some grounding black sesame oil.

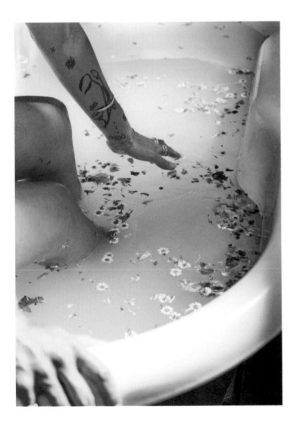

FOOD IS MEDICINE

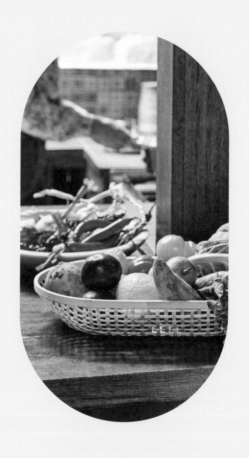

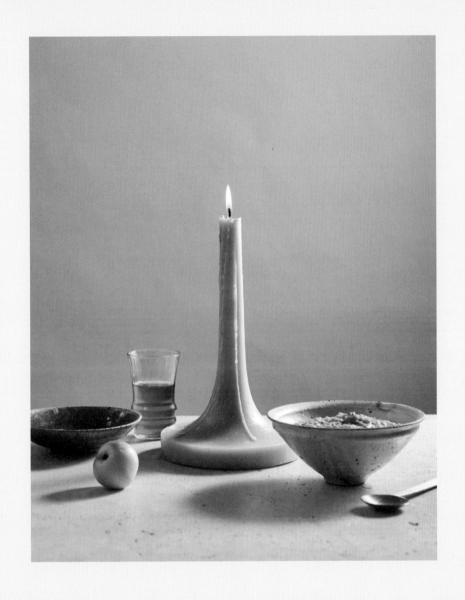

The fundamentals of the Ayurvedic diet

The Ayurvedic diet has one mission in mind – to provide the body with nutrition to sustain energy while both preventing and healing disease through delicious, wholesome, plant-based foods straight from Mother Nature's garden.

Ayurveda recognises several factors that determine the effect food has on our body, such as the strength of our digestive power (Agni), the energy we impart while cooking and eating, the time of day we have our meals, the compatibility of food groups, the balance of the elements within our meal, the heating or cooling effect our food has on our constitution, the spiritual and life-force energy of our produce, the importance of freshly cooked, seasonal meals and how to support digestion through medicinal spices, aperitifs and digestifs.

This is the art of eating well to support our physical, mental, emotional and spiritual wellbeing while reducing our impact on the planet and all of its creatures.

Ayurveda is not fixated on micro- and macronutrients or calorie counting; far removed from food fads that come and go, it is about considering a number of factors. These include eating locally grown organic and seasonal foods within a timeframe that supports digestion, and honouring the fundamentals of age-old cooking practices that spark Agni (digestive fire) and contribute to the elimination of toxic residue (Ama), while supporting every cell in your body.

Also important are the physical and spiritual qualities of your produce and how these affect your mental disposition. This may sound a little overwhelming at first but all of the principles make sense and will resonate deeply with you as you begin to implement them in your kitchen.

This is about educating yourself on what you can do to give yourself the best opportunity for vibrant health while creating a rhythm in the kitchen that makes you want to explore and experiment more and more. Cooking is a sacred ritual that should bring you joy, health and vitality.

So what does a healthy diet look like?

Like all facets of Ayurveda, what is right for one is not right for all, so it's about recognising your constitution, but most importantly it's about which elements or Dosha are aggravated, and integrating the qualities of the counter-balancing Dosha to restore harmony. The food we eat should not only nourish our body, but our mind and emotions as well – meaning that everything we consume has a spiritual effect on us also. Ayurveda also has a set of Golden Guidelines (see page 122) that influence not only how we cook but how we eat.

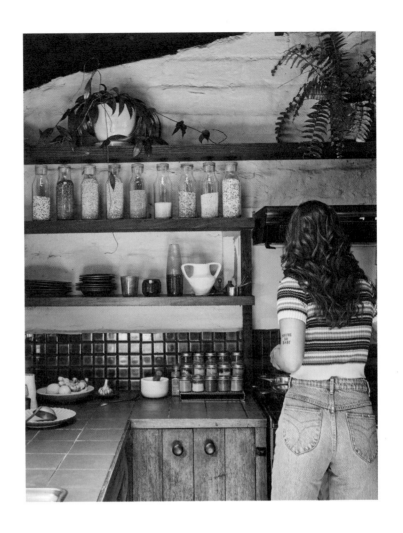

Generally, an Ayurvedic diet is largely plant-based, consisting of fruit, vegetables, nuts, seeds, legumes, grains, oils, herbs and spices. These foods contain the most life-force energy, or Prana.

The digestive fire (Agni)

Our ability to process everything we consume from our environment is a reflection of the internal strength of our digestive power. 'Agni' is the Sanskrit word for 'fire' and is known as the manifestation of the metabolism with its ability to break down and transform everything we are exposed to, including food, thoughts, emotions and the impressions we take in via our senses – our eyes, ears, nose, tongue and skin.

Ayurveda does not believe that you 'are what you eat', rather it believes that you 'are what you digest'.

This means that even if you have a perfect diet, if your digestive power (Agni) is not strong, you simply can't break down or absorb the nutrients from your food, which leads to the accumulation of toxins (Ama) from the decay of food rotting, which are then transported through the blood and cause problems for the liver, gut, skin and all other organs.

Responsible for our digestive function, Agni influences the assimilation of nutrients, the effectiveness of our senses and our mental capacity, which intertwine to reflect our overall state of wellbeing. Anyone who experiences sluggish digestion, acid reflux or any digestive issues is limiting themselves from the full experience of life and liberation from disease.

As the gut is the home of digestion, it is believed to be the largest breeding ground for disease when not functioning properly. Ayurveda considers poor digestion to be the basis for disease to manifest.

What negatively affects Agni?

o Mental health issues (first and foremost) such as stress, negative emotions, unrelieved trauma, depression, anxiety and low self-esteem.

o Poor lifestyle choices including lack of exercise and self-care, and abuse of the senses.

o Insufficient nutrition including a largely cooling diet with icy water, cold drinks, smoothies, ice cream, cooling foods like bitter vegetables cooked without appropriate spices, or raw foods that are very hard to break down.

o Dampening foods such as leftovers, food with no flavour or Prana (life force), long-life products and food with no nutritional value.

As Agni is associated with the Fire element, which is responsible for transformation within the body, it works in alignment with the sun's energy. Just as the day moves from dark to light, then back to dark, so too does our Agni, beginning with lightness in the morning, high intensity at midday and withdrawal back into darkness at night. This is a great tool for understanding your digestive power. Breakfast and especially dinner are not ideal times to consume heavy meals, as Agni is at its lowest. Lunch, in alignment with the midday sun, is the optimum time to have your biggest meal of the day so that your body has time to process and digest before stimulating foods can begin to interfere with your sleep.

The easiest way to decipher whether something is going to ignite or dampen Agni is by visualising a small burning fire within the stomach and asking yourself, 'Will this stoke the fire or put it out?' Obviously pouring a cold liquid onto a flame will instantly put out the fire; on the other hand, adding more heating elements like spices and cooked foods will help to keep the fire blazing.

Tools to support Agni:

o Avoid cold or cooling foods/drinks in excess.

o Favour cooked foods over raw.

o Drink room-temperature or warm water.

o Infuse herbal teas into your day such as ginger or CCF tea (page 130 also see Medicinal teas, page 180).

o Spices increase Agni by stoking the fire. They also aid digestion and the absorption of healthy nutrients (see Pantry essentials, page 126).

o Introduce an Agni-building aperitif prior to eating to stimulate digestion, as well as post-meal digestives (see page 130).

o Don't overeat! Too much food in the stomach dampens Agni and turns into waste, causing gas and bloating. It also promotes excess acid in the stomach, which causes reflux and indigestion. Cup your two hands together with fingers touching; that's how much food your body needs per meal.

o Make lunch your largest meal of the day, with breakfast and dinner being the smallest/lightest.

o Eat consciously. The best way to get the most out of your meal is to really sit with it and enjoy every mouthful. When we are preoccupied with conversation, TV, working etc. while we eat, our body is trying to focus on too many things at once and gets distracted from digesting properly.

This habit prevents our brain from recognising how much food we've consumed, so it takes more to get that 'satisfied' feeling.

o Movement, especially yoga and pranayama (breathing exercises), is very beneficial for circulating new energy and igniting Agni.

o Release negative emotion, as feelings of stress, fear, anxiety and sadness largely inhibit the function of the stomach and gut (see page 112).

o Adopt lifestyle practices such as meditation, which can help restore the body's homeostasis (natural state of balance), including the processes controlling digestion.

o Try sitting down and just eating; the flavours will become so much more intense and the satisfaction will come quickly.

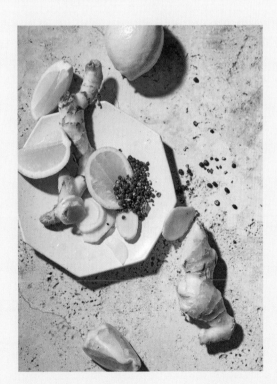

The Ayurvedic definition of 'health' is holistic and states that in order to embody true health and wellbeing:

'All Doshas must be working in harmony, we must possess a strong digestive fire (Agni), the waste systems (Malas) must be eliminating effectively, all tissues functioning, also the sense organs, mind and soul must be pleasant and happy.'

— SUSHRUTA
Vedic sage/physician

THE ROOTS

Hippocrates, the father of modern medicine, said, 'Let food be thy medicine and medicine be thy food' around 500 BC, thousands of years after the original Ayurvedic texts stated, 'Food is medicine when consumed properly'. Somewhere along the line, we lost sight of this fundamental aspect of diet and began to indulge in toxic food, which coincided with the array of health concerns we see today. We must remember that food is medicine, a healing force that is not to be underestimated. Having a healthy diet is the essence of disease prevention, a positive mental outlook, quality sleep and boundless energy, as well as being the key to longevity. By eating foods that are uniquely suited to your constitution and that address your imbalances, you are able to restore harmony on a daily, even hourly basis. You are your best adviser; if you are suddenly feeling hot-headed and stressed, take five minutes to brew a calming batch of chamomile, mint or fennel tea to cool you down. When we master the art of living, we are able to work with our body to treat symptoms before they have a chance to manifest further.

FINDING THE BALANCE

We possess the power to navigate through healthy food choices, as eating should be intuitive. When we are in balance, and in touch with our body, we naturally gravitate towards the forms of nutrition we are craving in order to restore balance, not to satisfy an addiction. When we crave things that are detrimental to our health, it's a very loud and clear message that there are some imbalances that need to be harmonised. The message is there if you dare to listen. When we are unsatisfied from a lack of nutritious food in our diet, we lean towards highly stimulating foods for that extra edge or quick fix, such as chocolate, sugar, spicy food and caffeine etc. The quality of the food we consume is fundamental to our overall sense of satisfaction. By consuming a well-balanced and wholesome diet, cravings for unhealthy snacks will begin to dissipate. Only you will know whether a food does or doesn't resonate with your internal needs, so pay attention to your response not only to the taste but also to the way in which your digestive system reacts.

EXPERIMENT WITH DIVERSITY

The principles of Ayurvedic cooking are by no means restricted to Indian cuisine. Once you develop a sense of the fundamentals and a relationship with the Six Tastes (see page 118), you can begin to implement these philosophies into almost any cuisine, from Mexican to Thai and beyond. If you have a Vata aggravation and you're in the mood for Italian, you can up your quantity of olive oil and swap the side salad for some sautéed baby carrots; a Pitta type might swap out the tomato passata for a cooling pesto sauce and side salad; and a Kapha type could opt for a lighter pasta made from semolina with baked broccolini. The possibilities are endless.

Did you know?

From a physical perspective, strong Agni means powerful immunity, energy, absorption, regular and consistent bowel function, strong bones, glowing skin, shiny hair, radiant eyes, the list goes on. From a mental perspective, Agni ignites joy, action, intelligence, brain function and a positive outlook on life. When Agni is hindered, feelings such as fear, anger, frustration and dissatisfaction may arise.

Gut health

As one of the most important functions of the human body, digestion and gut health are the ultimate physical pillars for health and wellbeing. So what exactly is the gut and why is it so important not only for our physical wellbeing but also our mental outlook?

The gut influences every aspect of our lives, from the obvious elements like the state of our digestion right through to our energy levels, the quality of our sleep, the function of our organs, even our innate level of happiness. The gut is responsible for absorbing nutrients and eliminating toxins or waste, so when it isn't functioning properly we can face issues with nutrient deficiencies and stored toxins. Both of these issues create a breeding ground for disease to exist, which is why gut health has become such a popular topic of conversation in the wellness community. Even modern science is now labelling the gut our 'second brain', as it houses so many of the cells that influence our mood, as well as a large per cent of the cells that make up our immune system, and controls the production of serotonin, also known as the 'happy hormone'.

Gut health extends much further than simply the state of our small and large intestines. It's vast and complex and should be a priority when it comes to obtaining health. Ayurveda takes a holistic approach, extending far beyond probiotics into the realms of mental health, the strength of our digestive fire (Agni), as well as a vast exploration of our diet and lifestyle practices.

DIGESTION

Remember that the most notable difference between the Western approach to gut health and Ayurveda's is the onus that Ayurveda puts not only on what we eat, but what we digest. This means that we can have the best diet under the sun, but if we are not able to digest the vast array of nutrients properly, then they are of no use to us and can actually become toxic as they begin to decompose. Ayurveda has a saying that it is 'better to have a bad diet and good digestion, rather than a good diet and bad digestion', which highlights exactly how important it is to support our digestive power. Hippocrates himself stated that 'all disease begins in the gut'. When our food is not properly digested, it becomes the toxic residue known as Ama. The build-up and accumulation of compounding Ama is seen as the root cause of most disorders. Ama is the by-product of anything that we eat – from fruit to meat – that remains within us, plaguing the gut and subsequently the rest of our organs. When our digestion is strong, we possess the ability to digest and absorb nutrients from everything we consume, so the ultimate intention is to strengthen Agni, which equates to supreme gut health.

ABSORPTION

There are several different stages throughout the process of digestion, beginning with our vision! That's right. Ayurveda considers digestion to include all of our five senses, which is why cooking our own meals is a great booster for our digestive power. As we experience the aroma of our food as it simmers away on the stove, our tastebuds become tantalised, leading our eyes and nose to send signals to our brain that food is on the way, which activates certain triggers to begin preparing for digestion.

The next stage begins in the mouth via the salivary glands. Our tastebuds tell our brain what's on the menu so that the brain can determine what is needed to break down the specific foods we are consuming. When we ingest anything, including medicine and supplements that are tasteless, it hits the stomach without this warning, and our body marks it as an 'intruder' and does its best to eliminate it as quickly as possible. Taste is absolutely vital in the process of digestion, which is why Ayurveda recommends the experience of taste even when taking herbs and medicine. It is fundamental to our body's ability to decipher what is good for us, what is not and how to get the most out of whatever we're consuming.

Once our meal makes it to our stomach, it is further broken down and sent off to the small intestine, which is where most of the assimilation of nutrients takes place, as they are absorbed into the bloodstream. Any leftover matter makes its way through the large intestine on its way to be eliminated with an assortment of other cells the body is no longer in need of.

The strength of our Agni determines how efficiently this innate flow traverses the landscape of our internal environment and whether our food becomes our medicine or our poison.

FOOD INTOLERANCES

Our modern world is experiencing a rate of food intolerances and allergies like never before. Civilisation has evolved through the consumption of foods such as wheat, nuts and dairy, yet a growing number of children born today are fatally allergic to these age-old nutrients. The problem is not just the foods themselves, but the processes they are subjected to and the chemical additions that infest them. Most crops are now heavily sprayed with chemicals and drastically altered from their original state, which is causing a lot of health problems. This has placed great strain on modern families that live in fear of their children having a potentially lethal reaction, and has also created a massive inconvenience for anyone trying to dine out. Western medicine's solution is to eliminate the offenders and work your life around a very restrictive and sometimes impossible dietary confinement. Ayurveda's approach is simple – increase your digestive power so that your body can tolerate all foods, and consume high-quality produce that is organically grown and non-GMO. Of course, this entails a period of avoiding triggering foods, but this is a short-term solution while you build Agni and eventually start reintroducing foods and working with the subtle language of your body to reintegrate them into your life. If you are suffering from food intolerances, we have to ask the question – how strong is your digestive fire and what are the sources of your food? In the West we are often given medication to control or numb the symptoms of a problem rather than looking at the root cause and eliminating it entirely or simply improving the digestive function. Rather than allowing external factors to control and shape our human experience, we must come back to our internal source and build our resilience so that we remain in control of our body and our life.

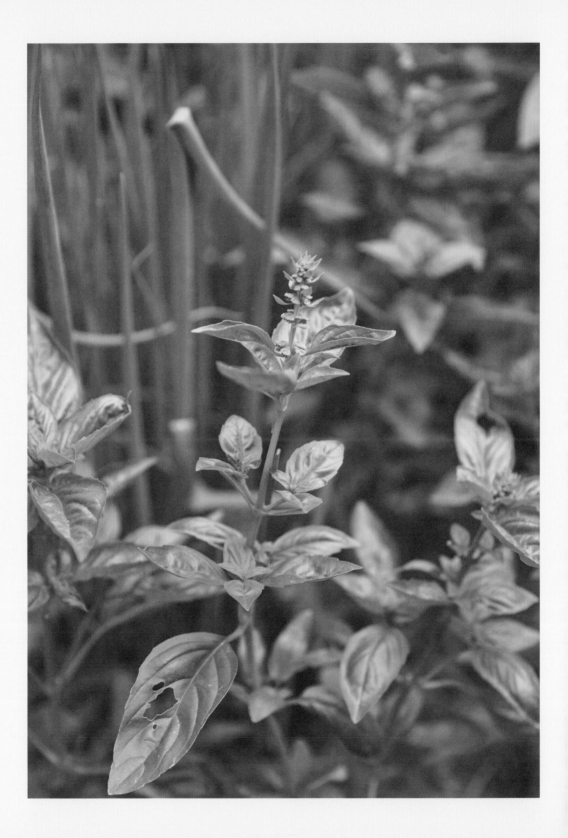

Life-force energy (Prana)

Known as life-force energy, Prana is the element of medicine that lives within food. Prana is life-giving, health-promoting and an amazing agent for healing. Prana means to be alive, to eat foods that are flooded with nutrients and hold the potential to give life.

When we can walk into our garden, pluck an apple off the tree and bite right in, that apple is still alive, meaning that all of the nutrients that live within it are still singing and ready to flood your body with the nectar of life. When that apple was taken from a tree on another continent, outside of your local environment, sprayed with chemicals to keep it alive, then frozen for months on end while it traverses the seas to be stored in a supermarket warehouse, it is void of Prana. The nutrients that were giving it life while it was connected to the tree and earth have long gone. The sooner we can eat produce after it has been harvested, the more Prana it will contain. As meat comes from animals that have been killed, Ayurveda believes that it holds a negative or Tamasic (dormant) energy and is void of Prana. The most Prana-rich foods are Sattvic (pure) by nature and come from a plant source that is connected to the life-giving properties of Mother Nature.

Ayurveda operates under the ideology of Ahimsa, which is the philosophy of non-violence towards all living, sentient beings through the consideration of love first always. This way of living can be exercised within our thoughts and actions towards ourselves, others, the planet and all creatures with which we share this sacred land. In adopting this school of thought,

we should strive to extend love to everyone and everything while refraining from any negative or destructive behaviours; this includes the restriction of animal agriculture. Ayurveda does not condone the farming of animals, as this does not support the values of Ahimsa, nor does it impart Pranic energy into our diet. Outside of the energetic effects on the body, the meat industry is one of the largest contributors of harmful emissions into the environment. Buddhist monk Thich Nhat Hanh writes in his book *The World We Have: A Buddhist Approach to Peace and Ecology* that 'By eating meat we share the responsibility of climate change, the destruction of our forests, and the poisoning of our air and water. The simple act of becoming a vegetarian will make a difference in the health of our planet.'

As food must contain Prana in order for it to be able to nurture us, it is said that the better the quality of the food, the more potent the medicine. This means that organic produce, grown locally and in season, harvested from a nearby farm and consumed within a short period of time is believed to provide the ultimate source of nutrition. Prana flows through us, nurturing every cell in the body. When your food is alive, your skin, eyes, hair and nails will look and feel vibrant and alive.

Heating + cooling foods

Everything we consume has either a heating or cooling effect on the body, meaning that our diet can drastically influence our mood, digestion, circulatory system and body temperature. By nature, heat expands and cold contracts, meaning that heat promotes fluidity, moisture, movement and unctuousness, whereas cold restricts flow and sharpens rigidity. The inside of the body is almost like a gushing waterfall of endless rapids and rivers traversing several streams of nourishment; to keep these tides turning, it's important to provide plenty of hydration and promote circulation to avoid stagnation.

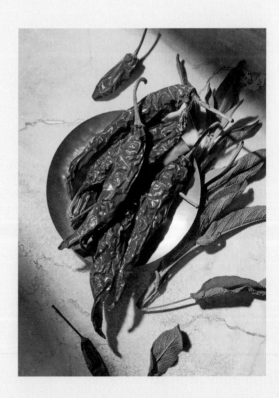

HEATING FOODS

Heating foods ignite Agni by adding fuel to the fire; they are stimulating, as they enliven our senses and invigorate our soul; they help to motivate and move us throughout the day; they inspire all of our bodily functions, especially digestion and blood flow, as well as lubrication of our joints; and they are the most beneficial to the body. Heating equals healing, as the promotion of the circulatory system, or blood network, sends fresh oxygen around the body, which allows it to heal and repair damaged cells and compromised tissues and eliminate dangerous invaders or bacteria. As with everything, there is always a fine balance that has the potential to be tipped over when heating foods are consumed in excess. Too much heat can contribute to anger, competitiveness, control, jealousy, insomnia and other heightened mood swings. This is easily avoided by monitoring your intake of stimulating substances such as hot spices, salt, sugar, caffeine and alcohol. Cooling foods, on the other hand, are much more subdued by nature. They are calming and can be a perfect antidote when there is too much heat in the body, but must be used with caution, as they can inhibit Agni and cause internal dryness.

COOLING FOODS

It is only when either our internal or external environment is excessively hot that cooling foods and substances have their place. Even then, it's better to try and cool down topically first before ingesting too many cooling substances. Rather than diving into a tall glass of iced water in the summer, try applying ice topically to the neck and temples, soaking the feet in a cool ice-bath, taking a cold shower, drinking room-temperature water with a cooling herb like mint, or chewing fennel seeds throughout the day. All of these approaches will help to bring your body temperature down without dampening Agni. Cooling substances are friends of Pitta, as they balance the Fire element. Kapha and Vata are cool by nature, so those with these Doshas should limit the amount of cooling substances in their diet.

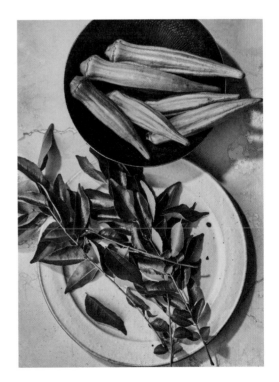

The Six Tastes

Everything we eat falls under one of the Six Taste groups – Sweet, Sour, Salty, Pungent, Bitter and Astringent – and each of these groups is associated with the Great Elements (Space, Air, Fire, Water and Earth), which either increase or decrease specific Doshas. By cultivating a relationship with the Six Tastes, you will intuitively be able to craft your diet to support your innate needs on a daily basis.

Taste	Elements	Dosha	Temp	Effect
Sweet (Grounding)	Water + Earth	V− P− K+	Cooling	Grounding, nourishing, building; promotes weight gain, longevity, strength, healthy bodily fluids and tissues. Balances Vata
Sour (Alertness)	Earth + Fire	V− P+ K+	Heating (moderate)	Moistens, stimulates thoughts, emotions, appetite, digestion and elimination. Balances Vata
Salty (Stimulating)	Water + Fire	V− P+ K+	Heating (mildest)	Stimulating, hydrating, improves digestion, detoxifying, cleanses tissues, boosts absorption. Balances Vata
Pungent (Spicy)	Fire + Air	V+ P+ K−	Heating (hottest)	Stimulates digestion, increases Agni, improves appetite, clears sinuses, stimulates blood circulation and cognitive function, heightens the senses. Balances Kapha
Bitter (Calming)	Air + Space	V+ P− K−	Cooling	Highly detoxifying and pacifying of infection, weight reducing, calms mental distress, defuses fire; anti-inflammatory/antiviral/antibacterial. Pitta and Kapha pacifying
Astringent (Drying)	Air + Earth	V+ P− K−	Cooling (mildest)	Light, drying, cooling, anti-inflammatory, mentally purifying; stops bleeding. Pitta and Kapha pacifying

The Sweet taste is composed of the elements Earth + Water, known as Kapha Dosha. When a person consumes anything from the Sweet category, they are increasing their intake of Kapha. If they are already a Kapha type, or have a Kapha aggravation (excess weight, water retention, flu-like symptoms such as mucus/congestion, allergies, depression etc.), they are likely to be contributing to their Kapha aggravation, so these foods are best replaced with more of the Pungent, Bitter and Astringent tastes, which burn off and pacify the moisture of the Kapha Dosha.

Avoid	Examples
If trying to lose weight or having difficulty with digestion. Kapha aggravating	Wheat, rice, dairy, cereals, grains, eggs, meat, dates, prunes, bananas, mangoes, melons, beetroot, sweet potato, carrots, pumpkin (winter squash), olives, nuts, all sweeteners, licorice root
If feeling stressed, aggressive or hot-headed. Pitta aggravating	Lemons, limes, grapefruit, tomatoes, vinegars, butter, cheese, sour cream, yoghurt, pickled and fermented foods, tamarind, wine
If feeling stressed, aggressive or hot-headed. Pitta aggravating	Sea salt, Himalayan salt, rock salt, sea vegetables (seaweed, kelp etc.) tamari, cottage cheese, celery, black olives, processed foods
If overly stimulated, critical, hot-headed, suffering from insomnia or an overactive mind. Pitta aggravating	Hot spices like chilli, cayenne, paprika, asafoetida (hing), black pepper, hot peppers, radish, ginger, onions, garlic, mustard
In excess if suffering from Vata aggravation or extreme dryness in the body	Herbs like coriander (cilantro), mint, dill etc., all green leafy vegetables, artichokes, turmeric, most herbal teas
In excess if suffering from Vata aggravation or extreme dryness in the body such as constipation, gas or light period	Unripe bananas, green grapes, pomegranates, cranberries, green beans, cruciferous vegetables, raw vegetables, wheat, rye, beans, popcorn

Food combining

Conscious food combining could be your saving grace when it comes to effortless digestion, improved energy and sleep, clearer skin and deeper nourishment, and could make a huge improvement to your overall health. The concept is simple – some foods digest well together, others do not.

Ayurveda finds beauty in simplicity – keeping the variety of ingredients in a meal to a minimum while using spice and aroma to impart taste. Our tastebuds have been hugely altered since the introduction of intense sweeteners and artificial flavours, enticing us to crave such bold flavour profiles. By consuming an Ayurvedic diet, you will be able to refine and recalibrate your palate to enjoy the robustness of earthy delights without the need for extreme flavours that knock you off the edge of your seat.

The art of food combining can be a little intimidating at first, especially considering that most of the classic dishes in the West are wildly incompatible, but once you get the hang of it, your digestive system will thank you and you'll know how to navigate your way through a meal without disturbing the delicate balance that lives within. What a lot of people mistake as food allergies are often just reactions to improper combinations of food. When incompatible food groups hit the stomach, the body begins the process of digesting one, which can be vastly different to the process the other food would undergo, and therein lies the problem. The stronger your Agni is, the more equipped you are to handle difficult combinations, so pay attention to how you feel after each meal and take this into consideration.

Acquiring this knowledge is a key component in making healthy choices for yourself and your future. Try not to think of this as a set of black and white rules, but rather as tools you can use to improve your digestion in general. Of course, you're not expected to live by them on every occasion, but armed with this wisdom you have the full potential to create a life for yourself free from disease and discomfort.

Did you know?

Fruit is high in natural sugar and is naturally metabolised very quickly, providing nutrients for the brain and energy for the body. If fruit is consumed with or after any other food, let's say a piece of toast, the process of digestion grinds to a halt as the body takes its time to metabolise the bread while the fruit is left to rot and decompose, which then creates gas and bloating, and even spikes in insulin, which can result in weight gain. This is where a lot of the fear around fruit sugars comes from. But if fruit is consumed on its own, away from other foods, it is nature's candy and provides a plethora of wonderful nutrients for the entire body.

Food	Compatible with	Incompatible with
Fruit	Similar fruits (berry medley, oranges and grapefruit, or apples and pears)	Everything else, including fruit salad of all varieties and every other food
Lemons	Most foods in a small quantity	Cucumber, tomatoes, milk, yoghurt
Melon	Other melons	All foods
Vegetables	Other vegetables, grains, beans, seeds, nuts, cheese, yoghurt, eggs, fish, meat	Fruit, milk
Nightshades	Other vegetables, grains, beans, seeds, nuts, fish, meat	Fruit, cucumber, all dairy (milk, yoghurt, cheese)
Beans	Grains, vegetables, nuts, seeds	Fruit, milk, cheese, yoghurt, eggs, fish, meat
Grains	Beans, vegetables, other grains, seeds, nuts, yoghurt, cheese, fish, meat	Fruit
Butter, Ghee	Grains, vegetables, stewed fruit, beans, nuts, seeds, eggs, fish, meat	N/a – opt for ghee in cooking
Cheese	Grains, vegetables	Fruit, beans, eggs, milk, yoghurt, fish, meat
Milk*	Porridge, dates, almonds	All other foods, especially salt, bananas, melons, citrus, fish, meat
Yoghurt	Grains, vegetables	Fruit, nightshades, beans, milk, cheese, eggs, fish, meat
Eggs	Grains, non-starchy vegetables	Fruit, potatoes, all dairy (milk, cheese, yoghurt), beans, fish, meat

Must always be boiled

The Golden Guidelines for eating

Think of cooking as if you are creating art. There should be colour, texture, creativity and love; it should ignite the senses and stimulate the soul. By cooking consciously, being fully present in the kitchen and directing all of your attention and energy into what you are creating, your food will be infused with the cosmic vibration of love. When a meal has been lovingly, patiently and tenderly prepared, you really can taste the difference. This is what makes a home-cooked meal or nanna's cookies so special. As you are not only feeding your tastebuds, ensure that your meal is a visual feast that can be enjoyed by your other sense organs that contribute to digestion. Express gratitude, even in silence; take a moment before you eat to give thanks for the nourishment you are about to receive and welcome it into your body.

Ayurveda urges you to listen to your body, to develop a felt language with yourself that allows you to tap in and connect with the experience of your meal. Does it make your cells feel alive or does it strip you of energy? Does it make your tummy gurgle and gassy or does it pass through you with ease? How are your eliminations affected by what you've eaten? These are all practical messages that can give you a clear understanding of what foods do or don't agree with your body. If you are reacting to the foods recommended for your Dosha, it's important to build your Agni rather than just avoiding particular food groups, as this can lead to nutrient deficiencies.

THE GUIDELINES

o   Try to eat between sunrise and sunset while your Agni is alive, in alignment with the sun's energy.

o   Your food should be life-giving, seasonal, local, fresh and tasty.

o   Think and plan ahead. Make sure your pantry is always stocked with fresh spices and dried goods to avoid quick fixes on junk or fast food. Also roasting, toasting and/or soaking seeds, nuts, grains and legumes makes them easier to digest, so factor this in to your meal preparation.

o   Fresh is best. Ideally we would cook every meal from scratch but in the modern world this can be a challenge. Try to avoid anything cooked more than a day or two ago, reheat slowly on a low heat, jazz up leftovers with fresh ginger and black pepper to stimulate digestion, and resist the temptation to add fresh produce to leftover food.

o   Buy in bulk whenever possible to avoid single-use plastic. There are shops popping up all over the world that encourage you to bring your own jars or use paper bags to skip the plastic altogether. Store your produce in glass jars away from direct sunlight to extend its shelf life.

o   Avoid processed foods as much as possible. This includes anything altered from its original state. These offenders usually come in plastic and include ingredients that seem impossible to pronounce. Opt for fresh produce over canned, jarred or frozen varieties that hold little or no Prana.

o   Choose organic whenever possible. Or even better – grow your own. Gardening is seen as the perfect antidote and preventative for depression, as it is naturalistic, grounding and earthing.

- Pay attention to your energy. Your thoughts, feelings and conversations pervade your cooking. Avoid arguments, negative thoughts or discussing illness/disease while cooking and eating.

- Work from a blank canvas. Make sure your kitchen is clean and tidy before you begin. Do as many dishes along the way as possible so you don't have to come back to chaos after you have eaten. Try to prepare your ingredients individually before you turn on the heat, to reduce the stress of trying to chop and cook at the same time.

- Cook healthy, warm and unctuous (moist) foods (as opposed to raw) that respect the laws of food combining (see page 120) and incompatibilities.

- Avoid taste testing while cooking, as this triggers the process of digestion prematurely. Learn to trust your instincts and develop a sense of intuition in the kitchen. Pay attention to the colour and aroma as you cook, then when you do eat, make a mental note of any alterations you need to make next time.

- Don't depend on recipes alone; learn to cook for your palate and needs. Be creative and implement Ayurvedic principles into the dishes you know and love.

- Cooking and eating in a harmonious atmosphere turns food into nectar. Express gratitude, be present and taste your food fully – and avoid doing anything else while eating! Don't eat too fast or too slow. Chew your food so that you can press it between your tongue and the roof of your mouth; anything too formed will not be digestible.

- Don't eat until your last meal has been digested and you actually feel hungry! By snacking, grazing and eating prematurely we are inhibiting the digestion of our last meal. Ayurveda recommends a period of four hours between meals and doesn't suggest snacking unless you do very physical work.

- Eat an appropriate portion, measured by cupping your two hands together; we don't want to aim for feeling 'full'. We need to leave a quarter of our stomach empty for digestion.

- Eat for your body type and prioritise any imbalances or aggravations that need pacifying. Include the Six Tastes in each meal.

- Avoid drinking too many liquids during meals and for 30 minutes either side of eating, as they can dilute stomach acids needed for digestion.

- Don't be afraid of natural sugars like honey, agave, rapadura, jaggery, maple syrup etc.; in the right quantities, they are medicine for the body and food for the brain, but be sure never to heat honey (see page 132) – only use it raw!

- Natural fats contained in oils, ghee, nuts and avocado are also essential for the body and contribute largely to the health and longevity of the skin. Fats provide moisture that inhibits the signs of ageing.

- Cooking should be an adventure, not a chore! Have fun, get creative and enrich your meals with loving vibrations.

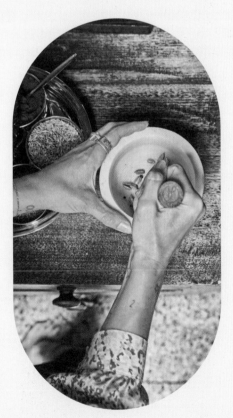

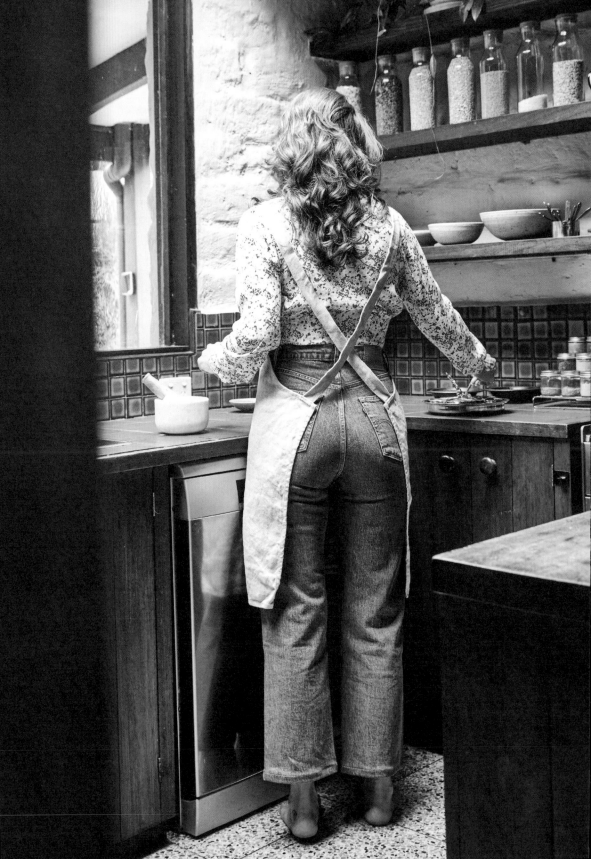

Your Ayurvedic kitchen

The kitchen is valued as the heart of the home, the central point where families come together and create loving meals to nurture and nourish the body, mind and spirit.

Honour the sanctity of the kitchen by ensuring that it is clean, uncluttered and organised, assisting with the flow of cooking – as in, the knives should be kept close to the chopping board, the spices nearby (but not above) the stovetop, and the serving bowls/plates within arm's reach. You want everything to be right where it should be, when you need it. It's best to make sure everything is ready to go and the drying-up rack is empty before you begin preparing your next meal.

As a science that dates back thousands of years, Ayurveda embraces raw, earthy materials that embody the Five Great Elements to complement and enhance the ingredients we use in our meals. Every material is seen to possess a certain energy, so you want to ensure you have good quality kitchenware for preparing, serving and storing your food. Setting up your kitchen is simple, as most of the tools are the age-old basics you probably already have, and will allow you to declutter by removing some of the appliances you may no longer need. Ayurveda prefers working with our hands rather than electric appliances, giving it a more romantic sensibility. Grinding flours and spices with a mortar and pestle, kneading dough with our bare hands, even eating our meals by hand, allows us to fully connect with our food and become part of the physical journey of loving preparation. The use of electric devices disturbs the cellular structure of food and should be avoided wherever possible. Plastics contain nasty chemicals that can leach into food, so should also be avoided.

Setting up your kitchen, you'll need:

o Various pots and pans, preferably with lids:

> Stainless steel conducts heat without interfering with the food.

> Enamel protects the energy of the food.

> Cast iron enriches the iron content in food and is favoured by Ayurveda.

> Copper conducts the most heat of all metals and is antibacterial.

> Clay is the richest source of earth and the most grounding.

o Stainless steel or glass mixing bowls

o Wooden bowls

o Glass containers

o Measuring spoons and cups (preferably copper or stainless steel)

o Wooden rolling pin

o Serving spoons and ladle

o Stainless steel colander

o Mortar and pestle

o Sharp knife

Pantry essentials

Ayurveda values fresh produce, fruit and vegetables, seeds and nuts, grains, beans, legumes and pulses, oils, herbs and spices. Fresh is best, so pay attention to the use-by dates, store them in glass away from sunlight and avoid anything with chemicals or preservatives.

The great news is that most of the Ayurvedic pantry essentials are very affordable and have a long shelf life, meaning that you can nourish yourself regardless of your budget and will always have enough in the cupboard to whip together a meal at the drop of a hat.

Most of these ingredients are now available at supermarkets, organic grocery stores, bulk-food shops, local markets, online or at Asian/Indian supermarkets. Explore what's on offer and opt for the brightest and freshest looking produce.

OILS

The starting point for many dishes, oils contain essential fatty acids that keep both the internal and external body moist, unctuous, lubricated and glowing. In recent times, fats have been taboo, which has been a leading cause of the common Vata aggravation we see in women today, including dryness in the colon, dry skin, premature ageing, cracking, dry joints and arthritis. Oils can prevent and help heal all of these conditions. Be aware, though, that certain oils are heat sensitive and can become volatile and carcinogenic when they exceed their smoke point, so are best used raw. Get to know which oils are better for cooking and which should be left for dressing.

o **Ghee:** Ayurveda's golden nectar, ghee is the supreme favourite with countless uses but is famously used in cooking. Also known as clarified butter, it undergoes a process that removes most of the lactose, casein and milk solids that people with dairy intolerances struggle with, so it is a much more digestible form of butter. Ghee is not sensitive to heat, making it the perfect cooking oil. Ghee has Sattvic (pure) properties with an innate intelligence, known as Prabhava, for healing and repairing the body. It aids lubrication of the bodily tissues and plays a big role in the transportation of toxins out of the body. Ghee is also said to promote memory and intelligence, and to support Agni. Due to its high fat content, Kapha types should not use ghee in excess and, of course, anyone with a solely plant-based diet (vegan) should avoid it.

o **Coconut oil:** Perhaps the next best thing to ghee, and suitable for vegans, coconut oil is rich in nutrients for both the internal and external body. Coconut oil is also suitable for cooking, but be aware that it has a cooling effect on the body, so Vata and Kapha types shouldn't use it in excess. It is a favourite for Pitta types and makes for a good summer oil.

o **Toasted sesame oil:** Used largely for its distinctly nutty aroma, sesame oil can handle some heat but is best suited for use in marinades, sauces and noodle dishes. A good source of calcium for strong bones, teeth, nails and hair. Kapha types should avoid in excess.

o **Olive oil:** A versatile oil renowned for its nutritional content, it is best kept raw to preserve its flavour and internal cleansing properties.

o **Avocado oil:** Dubbed the 'beauty oil' due to its contribution to healthy skin and hair, this oil is also best kept raw to preserve its abundance of vitamins, minerals and magnesium.

SPICES

Known as 'Nature's medicine cabinet', for centuries spices were more expensive than gold because of their medicinal value. Spices add colour, flavour and aroma to any dish while enriching them with therapeutic value and boosting Agni to assist with digestion, absorption and the assimilation of nutrients. Most spices are high in fibre, minerals, vitamins and antioxidants. By developing a relationship with spices, you can intuitively work with your body to harmonise imbalances that arise daily and seasonally. Learn to respect the subtle energies of spices and ensure you are using them appropriately, as they can be a source of imbalance if used excessively. Each spice has its own unique flavour profile and inspires specific shifts in the body that can be drying, cooling, heating or stimulating and may have the adverse reaction to that which your body needs. Use this knowledge and your intuition to navigate your way through the healing powers of the spice kingdom.

o **Ajwain:** The underdog of the spice world, it can be tricky to find but is well worth the mission. Ajwain has a flavour profile likened to oregano or thyme, which makes it easy to integrate into Italian dishes. It is known for its ability to support digestion, dispel gas, heal an upset stomach, especially during pregnancy or for babies, treat respiratory conditions, reduce pain, remove Ama, soothe migraines and even prevent premature ageing and hair from greying.

o **Asafoetida:** Also known as hing, this pungent resin provides a wonderful alternative to onion and garlic while helping your body 'digest what you can't digest'. This is a spice to be used in very small quantities and to be avoided during pregnancy/conception.

o **Black peppercorns:** Known as 'black gold', black peppercorns ignite Agni, kickstart digestion, aid in absorbing nutrients (especially those in turmeric), protect against cell damage, aid digestive issues and are full of antioxidants.

o **Cardamom:** A lovely sweet spice, cardamom has a distinctly floral flavour so is best reserved for sweet treats, breakfast meals and beverages. A digestive aid, it is also known for its ability to cleanse the lymphatic system.

o **Chilli:** A powerful heating spice responsible for sparking Agni, metabolic function, lymphatic drainage and boosting the immune system. Chilli should be avoided during the summer months and in all Pitta conditions.

o **Cinnamon:** Earthy, spicy and sweet, cinnamon is a must-have in all sweet dishes. Cinnamon is lovely and warming, reduces depression, boosts circulation, reduces pain and nausea, assists digestion and lubricates the joints, among other qualities. Pitta types should avoid it in excess.

o **Cumin:** Used as both a seed and in a ground form, cumin adds a distinctly spicy and earthy aroma to dishes. It is also favoured in Ayurveda for its endless abilities to aid digestion, absorption, metabolism, circulation and detoxification. It is especially healing for allergies, as it is heating and drying, and is also good for cramps and to support breast-milk production.

o **Curry leaves:** An edible alternative to the bay leaf, curry leaves add a beautiful woody aroma to the beginning of your dish while aiding digestion and supporting the liver.

o **Curry powder:** A blend of spices more subtle than garam masala, with lighter flavours like cumin, turmeric, coriander (cilantro) and fenugreek.

o **Fennel:** Perhaps the sweetest of spices, fennel tastes like licorice/anise and has a cooling effect on the body when experiencing Pitta/excess heat. Fennel is a palate refresher, aids digestion and removes bloating/gas.

- **Fenugreek:** A small shrub containing powerful maple-like sweet seeds and fragrant, bitter leaves. This plant is known to keep the signs of ageing at bay, heal digestive upset, assist those suffering from high cholesterol and diabetes, promote breast-milk production and is used topically in cosmetics.

- **Garam masala:** A famous spice blend, or 'churna', that utilises bold and pungent spices like cinnamon, peppercorns, coriander (cilantro), cumin, cardamom, cloves, nutmeg, bay leaves and fennel. This is a great spice to have on hand as a standalone mix for any curry dish.

- **Ginger:** Sweet and spicy, ginger is a powerhouse of healing goodness with anti-inflammatory and antibacterial properties, among others. Ginger is known to reduce nausea and any problems with indigestion while kickstarting Agni and enhancing detoxification; it also provides pain relief from injuries, inflammation and joint pain.

- **Garlic:** Famous for its potent zing, garlic is best saved for when your body needs it most – during infections, coughs and colds – for its antiviral, antifungal and antibiotic abilities. When used regularly, the power of its medicinal content is diminished and it can become overly stimulating. Onion is much the same, so Ayurveda leans towards leeks, spring onions (scallion) and asafoetida (hing) as alternatives.

- **Mustard:** Used mostly in its black seed variety, mustard offers a woody and nutty aroma to dishes while aiding digestion through its heating abilities. Mustard seeds are a powerhouse of nutrients, especially rich in calcium and selenium for strong bones. Yellow mustard seeds are lighter and slightly sweeter than the dark versions.

- **Paprika:** With similar properties to chilli, smoked paprika can impart a lovely woody aroma to meals – a great substitute for anyone missing the flavour of meat from their dishes.

- **Saffron:** The queen of red herbs, saffron infuses a warm tint to everything she touches and is renowned for her blood-cleansing abilities, which help to reduce skin conditions and flush out toxins while reducing pain, assisting with urinary disorders and aiding absorption.

- **Turmeric:** Revered all over the world for its anti-inflammatory, antibacterial and antioxidant properties, turmeric is an excellent support for the liver as a blood purifier, assisting with detoxification and aiding the immune system and gut. This bright orange bulb offers a distinctly 'Indian' aroma to your food while dispelling acidity and inflammation from the body. Turmeric is heating and should not be used in excess by Pitta types. Always use it in combination with black pepper, which activates your ability to digest turmeric.

PULSES (BEANS, LENTILS, PEAS)

An absolute must-have pantry essential, pulses are an excellent source of fibre and protein, with protein needed to build and repair muscles and bones, and to produce hormones and enzymes. The general rule is: the larger the pulse, the longer the soak time and the harder it is to digest, so opt for lighter, split varieties when Agni is low.

- **Red split lentils:** If you have these in your cupboard, you can always make a meal! Simply boil them with some spices and you have a delicious dal ready in under 20 minutes. No soaking or preparation is required. These are the easiest pulse to digest, although they should be avoided in excess by Vata types and should be cooked with plenty of oil.

- **Mung:** A more robust pulse, these little green beans are packed with nutrients that assist cleansing and detoxification. They can be found in whole or split varieties – whole beans require soaking for 4 hours, whereas split ones only require 2 hours and are easier to digest. Mung beans are cooling, so are suitable in the summer and especially for Pitta types.

- **Chana dal:** Split chickpeas, these have a healthy dose of fibre and energy, making them a nice addition for bulking out soupy dishes or to stand alone in warm salads. They do require soaking overnight, as they can be difficult to digest.

- **Black-eyed peas:** Actually a small white bean

with a nutty earthy flavour, and a soft yet firm texture. They are packed with nutrients, are very satisfying and provide long-lasting energy. Soak overnight.

o **Black turtle beans:** The heaviest of the listed pulses, but packed with iron and folate, these dense, earthy beans provide long-lasting satisfaction. Perfect if you're in the mood for Mexican. Soak overnight.

GRAINS AND FLOURS

An essential ingredient in a holistic diet, whole grains are packed full of nutrients including protein, fibre, B vitamins, antioxidants, and minerals such as iron, zinc, copper and magnesium. It has been shown that a diet rich in whole grains reduces the risk of many serious diseases. Be aware of refined, processed and bleached grains, which are detrimental to health. Industrial farming and manufacturing processes have altered wheat over the years, which has resulted in excess gluten and intolerances that cause bloating and inflammation; there are plenty of alternative options if your body struggles to digest wheat.

o **Wheat:** Rich in essential nutrients, wheat is a necessary part of a holistic diet when Agni is strong. Look for high-quality organic whole wheat that has not been refined or processed.

o **Rice:** Adored by Ayurveda for its ability to provide fibre, nutrients and substantial energy while helping to reduce obesity. Opt for aged white basmati rice, as it is the most beneficial and easy to digest. Although brown rice has more nutrients, it is harder to digest and must be soaked first.

o **Barley:** Known for its ability to remove acidity and cholesterol from the body, barley is a great support for cleansing and for restoring balance. It is a hearty grain that provides nourishment and long-lasting satisfaction while being easy to digest. It is especially beneficial for Kapha, as it is

absorbing, cleansing and reducing.

o **Buckwheat:** Naturally gluten free, buckwheat is in fact a seed, with a nutty texture and earthy aroma that is rich in magnesium. It is fantastic in noodle form (soba) and is also ground into flour for baking and savoury dishes. Those with Pitta constitutions or aggravations should avoid it in excess due to its heating properties, and it is also best avoided if Agni is low, as it is quite heavy and can be hard to digest.

o **Quinoa:** A light and fluffy seed that is very easy to digest and full of protein and nutrients, quinoa can be used in porridge or as a lighter alternative to rice; it is also great ground into flour. Naturally gluten free.

o **Semolina:** The tip of wheat, semolina contains little gluten and is perhaps the easiest grain to digest, due to its lightness. It is fantastic in porridge for anyone with low Agni.

o **Oats:** Most oats are naturally gluten free but can be contaminated in the production process. Whole oats contain antioxidants that can improve cardiovascular health. Try soaking them overnight or toasting them lightly before cooking to make them easier to digest. Oats are a good source of energy for those with strong Agni. Avoid quick or instant oats.

o **Besan:** A favourite in Ayurvedic cooking, besan flour is derived from chickpeas and is also known as gram flour. It is great for savoury dishes, sweet treats and baking. Also use sparingly when Agni is low, as it can be hard to digest.

Did you know?

When preparing grains and pulses ensure grains and pulses are washed thoroughly before cooking them. Add them to a large bowl and cover with plenty of filtered water. Use your hands to stir the water through. Drain and repeat this process 2–3 times until the water runs clear. Finally, rinse in a colander under running water. Your grains and pulses are now ready to use.

Herbal digestives

Stimulating appetite and supporting digestion are some of the tools that can be used to improve Agni on a daily basis. If you can kickstart your digestive fire before you consume a meal, you are giving yourself the best chance to break down your food and absorb the nutrients from it while avoiding stomach upset or discomfort.

Before you eat, pungent tastes that contain the Fire and Air elements help to ignite Agni and create the space for digestion to occur; these are known as Deepana and can be likened to an aperitif.

'Aperitifs' to have before meals (Deepana):

o Ginger tea

o Grated fresh ginger with lime juice and cracked black pepper

o Chewing pippali (long black pepper) or a few pepper berries

o Trikatu – powdered herbal blend of pepper, pippali (long black pepper) and ginger

After meals, Pachana is taken, which can be likened to a digestif, as these promote stomach secretions that break down your meals and expel reflux, gas and bloating.

Digestives to have after meals (Pachana):

o Chewing fennel seeds

o Chewing cumin seeds

o Ginger tea

o CCF Tea: Cumin, coriander and fennel tea

CCF TEA

In a small pot, bring 1 teaspoon cumin seeds, 1 teaspoon coriander (cilantro) seeds and 1 teaspoon fennel seeds and 4 cups (1 litre/34 fl oz) of water to the boil. Continue to boil, uncovered, until the water reduces to half (2 cups [500 ml/17 fl oz]).

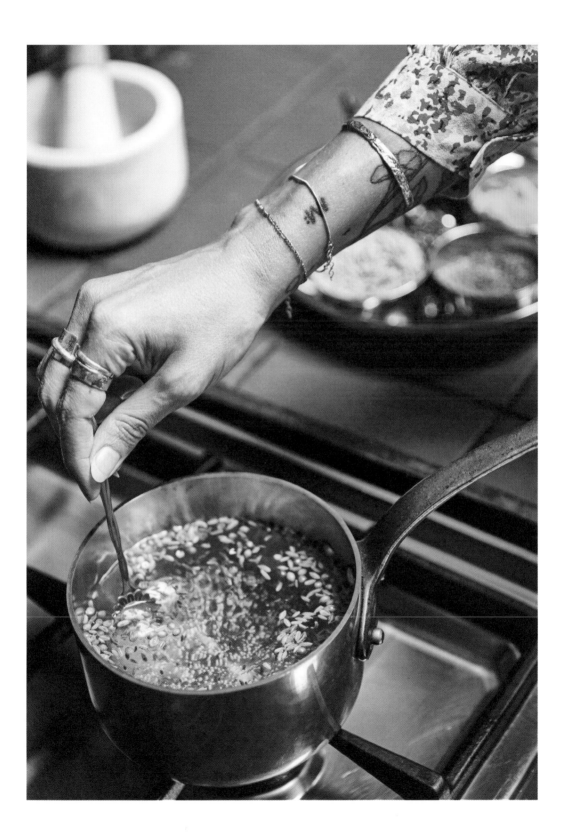

SWEETENERS

Natural sugar is the primary source of fuel for the body and the brain; without it we limit our ability to function and move through our day. When consumed in moderation, natural sugar activates the pleasure centre of our brain and releases a rush of dopamine, producing an immediate sensation of euphoria. Having a steady, appropriate amount of natural sugar in your diet is essential for healthy blood sugar levels, which provide energy and prevent cravings. Sugar only becomes a problem when it is processed or refined and exceeds the quantities your body requires. All sweeteners are rich in Kapha, so avoid in excess.

o Jaggery: Ayurveda's crown jewel when it comes to sweetening up everything from teas to treats. Derived from cane sugar juice, jaggery is not separated from the molasses, meaning that it still contains many essential nutrients and fibre, which makes it easy to digest and beneficial for the whole body! The lightest of the sweeteners.

o Coconut sugar: Derived from the coconut blossom or the sap of the tree, coconut sugar is higher in sucrose than jaggery, making it a little sweeter and more potent.

o Maple syrup: A great alternative to liquid honey, maple syrup is derived from the sap of the maple tree and is a great source of antioxidants and minerals like magnesium and zinc.

Honey is valued as a medicine rather than a food due to its highly antiseptic, antifungal and antibacterial healing abilities, as well as its high levels of antioxidants. A golden nectar dubbed 'nature's gift to mankind', honey has many medicinal benefits for both our internal and external body, assisting with the respiratory and digestive systems as well as skin conditions, metabolic function and weight loss, to name a few. Contrary to popular opinion, Ayurveda states that heating honey makes it poisonous. Why? Not only does heat weaken and destroy honey's enzymes, vitamins and minerals, it also converts it into a compound known as HMF, which becomes a non-homogenising glue-like substance that adheres to the mucous membranes and cells, clogging the pores of our internal channels, knowns as Srotas. Honey that has been heated is seen as toxic due to its inability to be digested, leading to the production of Ama (toxic residue); the European Union prevents the sale of honey that contains certain levels of HMF due to its levels of toxicity. The bottom line is that honey is a powerhouse of nutrition but should only be consumed raw. Most supermarket brands of honey have been heated and refined in the production process, so be aware of this and look for 'Raw Honey' on the label.

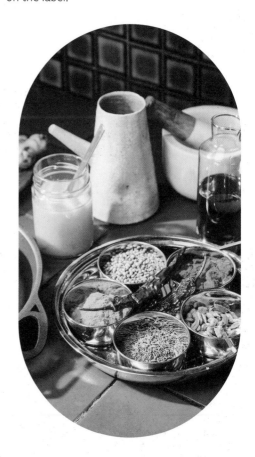

The science of rejuvenation (Rasayana)

In its purest, most literal form, 'Rasa' means taste. It is the experience we receive when our tastebuds and a meal unite for the first bite.

Rasa provides nourishment to all bodily tissues and is the basis of the immune system, so it's incredibly important to nurture your Rasa on a daily basis. From a physiological perspective, Rasa is likened to the plasma tissue that makes up the immune system and provides nourishment to every other tissue. If you are not nourishing your Rasa, you are abandoning your immune system and potentially crippling all of your other tissues, preventing them from living out their full potential. Rasa is largely responsible for the look and lustre of your skin, eyes, teeth, hair and nails, so by feeding Rasa you are preventing the signs of ageing. This is perhaps one of the best tools for achieving healthy, glowing skin that shines from the inside out.

Foods that nourish Rasa are known as Rasayanas and are largely made up of the Sweet Taste. Sweet foods are best consumed on an empty stomach, as they are metabolised very quickly on their own and provide wonderful nourishment for the whole body. These are foods we should consume for breakfast, avoiding them later in the day when there are heavier foods in the gut that prevent them from being metabolised as they should be. This is why skipping breakfast is not favoured in Ayurveda. The consumption of Rasayanas is all about nourishing the tissues, boosting energy and immunity, slowing the ageing process and bringing our body, mind and spirit back into a state of harmonious balance.

Forms of Rasayanas to be consumed between 6 am and 10 am:

Sip ½ cup (125 ml/4 fl oz) pomegranate or red grape juice with ½ cup (125 ml/4 fl oz) warm water.

Papaya with a squeeze of lime and fresh cracked black pepper.

1 teaspoon raw honey in 1 cup (250 ml/8½ fl oz) water (at room temperature).

Rasayana additions to porridge: dates, figs, currants, blanched almonds and walnuts.

Amla berry (found in Triphala herbal preparation).

Pick at least one of these items and have it daily to nourish Rasa.

Beyond the role it plays regarding the palate, Rasa is renowned as 'the essence of life'. It is what gives flavour to our very existence. This comes in several potent forms. It may be a delicious meal, but beyond that Rasa refers to sources of nourishment that inspire happiness, joy, laughter, sensuality and contentment – all of which are integral to health and wellbeing.

Rasa provides the fuel to motivate us to achieve our goals and also to sustain our energy levels, but just as a car needs the replenishment of fuel, so too do our bodies need Rasa to be replenished. An intense lifestyle combined with stress, deadlines, excessive work/exercise/socialising, sensory overload and poor lifestyle choices all dip into our reserve of Rasa, depleting our energy for the things that matter most. When we have insufficient Rasa, we can experience issues of poor immunity, low energy, chronic disease and other long-term health issues. One of the first signs of low Rasa appears with the signs of ageing. Have you ever wondered why some people appear to be forever youthful, whereas others begin ageing in their twenties? This is largely due to their level of Rasa. Think of Rasa as an internal juiciness that keeps us happy and healthy, and our skin plump.

The key aspect of understanding the value of Rasa is in comprehending the importance of happiness in your diet. Joy feeds the mind, body and soul with nourishment. A happy mind equates to a happy and healthy body. When we experience joy, we actually produce hormones that flood the body with goodness and also inspire deep healing while boosting the immune system. When someone is depressed (low in Rasa), their defences are also severely compromised and they become much more susceptible to disease. This knowledge only further solidifies the role that our mental health plays in our overall wellbeing.

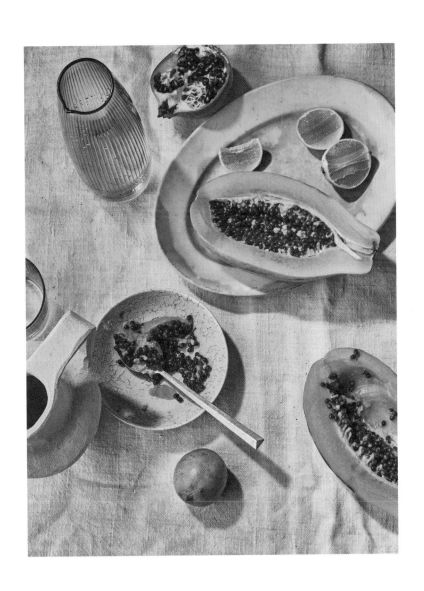

Diets for the Doshas

Ayurveda believes that what works for one doesn't necessarily work for the other, and similarly that what worked for you yesterday won't necessarily work for you today; this is why there is no blanket approach to this lifestyle and it's important to develop an understanding of your body and your needs and how to restore balance for yourself.

If you've experienced a sudden shift in mood or an emotional upset, your diet needs to support you through this turn while your body and mind 'digest' your experience. As complex, highly emotional and intelligent creatures, we are exposed to many highs and lows as we ride the tides of life, so it's important to tune in and listen to what your body is asking for. This is a powerful practice for staying connected with yourself and your innate needs. Once this language is established, the messages will become loud and clear, which can help you intuitively craft your ideal diet.

VATA DIET

The influence of the Air element in Vata creates a sense of lightness and dryness. By nature, Vata is cool, dry, rough and light. To balance these qualities, we need to introduce more grounding, nourishing, warming, oily, smooth and unctuous foods that will help to support Vata energy by drawing it back towards the earth, providing a stable base for grounding airy energy. Kapha is rich in Earth qualities that provide the perfect antidote for stabilising Vata. Kapha foods are heavy, moist, earth-bound foods such as oils, nuts, grains and root vegetables that are literally grown within the earth and therefore possess powerful grounding qualities. Pitta foods also provide the Fire element to heat up Vata's cold constitution and spark the digestive fire that can often become stagnant in Vata types, but these foods should not be used in excess as they can be drying for Vata. Pitta foods include spices like chilli, cayenne, cumin, ginger and turmeric as well as pineapples, olives, fermented foods, capsicums (bell peppers), onions and garlic. Creating an aromatic fusion of Kapha and Pitta foods will work to balance Vata and provide the energy to combat any physical limitations Vata types are prone to, such as constipation, flatulence, dry skin, weakness, joint pain, insomnia and forgetfulness.

Vata types or anyone with a Vata aggravation should avoid foods that are rich in Vata qualities, as they can lead to an over-abundance of Vata attributes. Vata-rich foods are drying by nature and include cruciferous vegetables, brussels sprouts, cabbage, kale, dried fruit, plain toast, crackers, popcorn and crisps, as well as foods cooked without juicy oils and nourishing sauces. To pacify Vata, opt for cooked grains, root vegetables, stewed fruit, nuts and seeds, warm drinks and spiced milk. Eat small meals regularly to support digestion, chew your food and be present while eating.

Signs of excess Vata:

o Physical: dry skin, premature ageing, thinning of hair, brittle bones, stiffness, cracking joints, constipation, flatulence and internal dryness.

o Mental: anxious, forgetful, scattered thoughts, distracted, trouble sleeping and finishing tasks.

PITTA DIET

The heat of the Fire element ensures Pitta types are always active and energetic, trailblazing their way through life with gusto and momentum. By nature, Pitta is hot, oily, moist and sharp. Introducing qualities that are cooling will help to calm the fire and prevent it from burning out of control, and this includes foods that are dry, mild and stabilising. Pitta is pacified by the Sweet Taste, which is grounding, and also the Bitter and Astringent Tastes, which dry out excess oiliness and moisture. These qualities are embodied in a blend of both Vata and Kapha foods like beans, potatoes, grains, oats, pasta, crackers, rice cakes, popcorn, seeds, fruit, root vegetables and fresh greens. Pitta types possess the strongest digestion, as the fire keeps Agni alive, meaning they can handle more raw and cooling foods than any other Dosha. Cooling foods are those that are quite literally cool in temperature like raw foods, fresh salads, juice, fruit and raw vegetables; those which have a cooling, energetic effect on the body such as limes, cucumber, apples, avocado, pomegranates, artichokes, broccoli, cauliflower, lettuce, bitter greens; fresh herbs like mint, coriander (cilantro), parsley, dill and neem leaves; dried spices like coriander (cilantro) seeds, fennel seeds, cardamom and cumin; coconut products such as coconut water,

oil or dried coconut; and legumes like adzuki beans, black-eyed peas, chickpeas, kidney beans, lentils and soybeans. Pitta has more freedom when it comes to pacifying its qualities, due to the strength of the internal fire, so familiarise yourself with cooling foods and the fire will be kept at bay.

As like increases like, when aiming to pacify Pitta, foods which are naturally heating or stimulating should be avoided. It is best to limit your intake of overly spiced, oily, sour, sharp and fiery hot dishes that include chilli, cayenne pepper, paprika, eggs, meat, hard cheeses, pineapple, olives, nuts, vinegar, fermented foods like sauerkraut, pickles, sour cream and heavy oils. While trying to impart calming energy, it is also best to minimise your exposure to caffeine and alcohol, which both add fuel to the fire. In an attempt to dry out some of the excess water, liquid and oiliness that comes from the Water element within Pitta, opt for more textured meals over soupy stews, such as baked root vegetables with chickpeas and rice versus watery dal. Make your mealtime a ritual; sit down and be present as you savour every mouthful and avoid allowing your thoughts to be distracted by work or stressful events.

Signs of excess Pitta:

o Physical: skin rashes, breakouts, sweating, burning sensations, itchiness, baldness, reflux, indigestion, loose stools/diarrhoea, high temperature and fever.

o Mental: hot-headed, angry, competitive, stressed, burnt out and uptight.

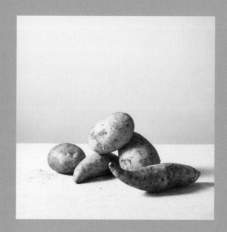

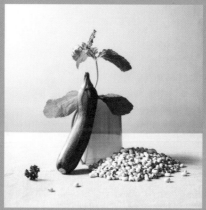

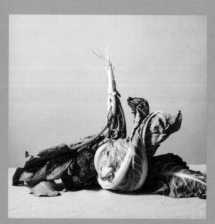

KAPHA DIET

The cool, calm nature of the Water element in Kapha keeps movement and mobility slow and steady. By nature, Kapha is oily, cold, heavy, smooth and regular. Heating qualities are required to give Kapha the kickstart it needs to get proactive and productive. Kapha is pacified by the Pungent, Bitter and Astringent Tastes and aggravated by the Sweet, Sour and Salty Tastes. Foods that are light, dry and warming help to counterbalance the heaviness of Earth energy while providing the spice of life necessary to combat stagnation and inspire action. A diet of freshly cooked warm whole foods that are light, dry, heating and well spiced serve Kapha's best interests. These foods include cruciferous vegetables and roughage like broccoli, cabbage, cauliflower, radishes, turnips, dark leafy greens, bitter greens (rocket [arugula], collard, dandelion greens etc.), bitter melon, apples, pomegranate, artichokes, eggplant (aubergine), basil, coriander (cilantro), dill, fennel, parsley; ginger, black pepper, cumin, cinnamon, garlic, paprika, and turmeric; crackers, rice cakes, popcorn, drying legumes such as adzuki beans, black-eyed peas, chickpeas, kidney beans, lentils and soybeans. Kapha thrives on simple meals that don't overburden their already earth-bound energy. Keep it light and you will be rewarded with more energy to power through your day.

Kapha-rich foods are best avoided, as they contribute to the accumulation of stagnant energy, leaving you unmotivated and uninspired. Do your best to minimise or avoid heavy and sweet foods like dairy (milk, ghee, cheese, yoghurt, ice cream), eggs, nuts, oils, zucchinis (courgettes), root vegetables, green grapes, oranges, grapefruit, pineapple, bananas, cakes, puddings, sweets, wheat-based pasta and bread, meat and fried foods. Also keep in mind that salty and sour foods have a tendency to aggravate Kapha. Opt for cooking with water rather than oil where possible. Due to the slow nature of Kapha, 2–3 meals per day is ideal with minimal snacking. Seek pleasure from every mouthful to get the satisfaction you so desire.

Signs of excess Kapha:

o Physical: weight gain, obesity, heaviness, shiny or oily skin, excess mucus and secretions, phlegm, respiratory disorders, sticky and heavy stools.

o Mental: lethargic, brain fog, unmotivated, jealous, highly emotional and depressed.

Utilise this ancient knowledge as stepping stones towards mastering your innate ability to become your own healer through listening to the subtle messages of your body. This is not about restriction; it's about respecting and honouring your body so that you are able to access a state of optimal health and wellbeing. It's the decisions we make on a daily basis that result in our mental disposition, so be wise with your choices and you will be rewarded.

	Vata	Pitta	Kapha
Favour	Cooked over raw Heating over cooling Oily over dry Soups over salads	Cooling over heating Dry over oily Nourishing over light Salads over soups Some raw foods	Cooked and raw Heating over cooling Dry over oily Light over heavy
Enjoy plenty of	Oils, cooked soft foods with warming spices, legumes and grains, citrus and sweet fruit, and root vegetables with a pinch of salt; add a side of something sour to your meals like a squeeze of lemon or vinegar and sauerkraut	Sweet fruit, grains, legumes, bitter greens, cooling herbs, salads, warm pakti bowls, some raw vegetables; add a squeeze of cooling lime to your dishes	Cooked cruciferous vegetables, bitter greens, lemons, light meals and textured pulses/beans, barley, healthy crackers and stimulating herbs and spices
Keep to a minimum	Raw and dry food like plain crackers and lentils/beans, wet greens, dry legumes, cruciferous vegetables, nutritional yeast, chilli and stimulants like coffee and alcohol	Stimulating foods like chilli and spicy herbs, citrus, fermented sour foods like tamari, pickles and sauerkraut; dairy, fast and processed foods, excess salt, stimulants like coffee and alcohol	Oils and fats, including coconut and avocado, nuts, sweeteners, olives, sour fruit, sweet fruit and root vegetables, pastries and desserts, excess salt, vinegar and dairy

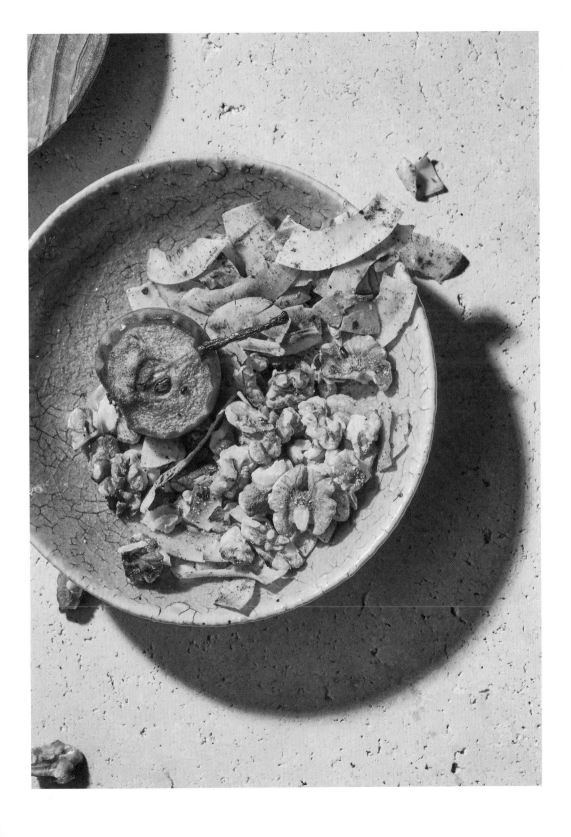

SOUL FOOD

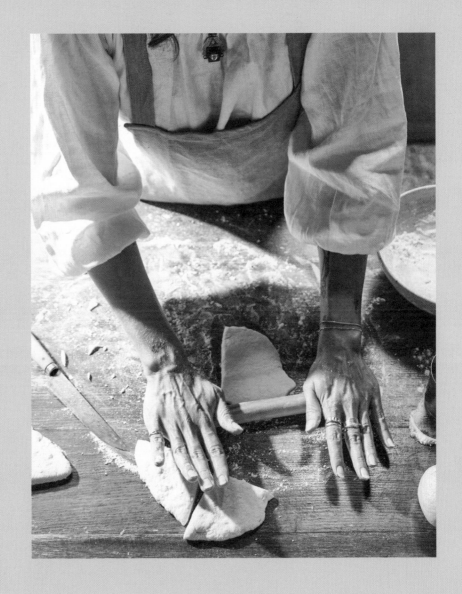

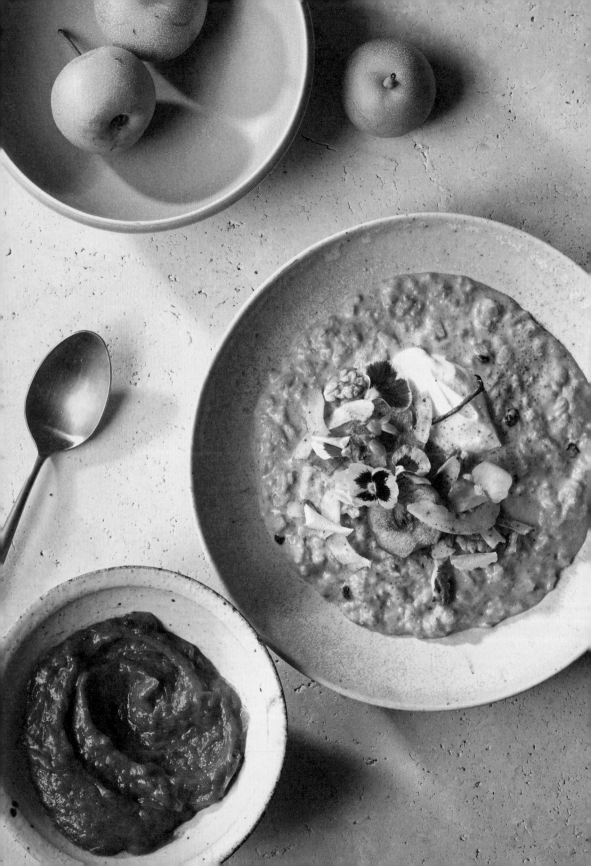

Grounding porridge with spiced seasonal fruit + nuts

This heart-warming and comforting porridge is the perfect dish to start the day, as it's light enough not to overburden your Agni first thing in the morning while providing a slow release of long-lasting energy. The element of Earth from the grains and fruit provides stability and structure to ground any nervous/flighty tension you may have towards your daily tasks.

Serves 1

Topping

1 teaspoon ghee or coconut oil

1 piece of seasonal fruit (apple, pear, banana, peach, plum, figs etc.)

1 tablespoon walnut pieces (or seeds/nuts of your choice)

1 tablespoon shredded coconut (optional)

pinch of cinnamon, for dusting

dollop of coconut yoghurt

Porridge

½ cup (50 g/1¾ oz) rolled (porridge) oats

1 cup (250 ml/8½ fl oz) milk of your choice

¼ teaspoon ground cinnamon

pinch of ground cardamom

1 teaspoon currants

1 teaspoon maple syrup or coconut sugar (optional), for serving

To serve (optional):
Zesty rhubarb & ginger compote (see page 146)

Heat the ghee or coconut oil in a cast-iron pan, add the fruit (face up) and cook for 1-2 minutes over medium heat.

Add the nuts and coconut to the pan and dust everything with cinnamon. Flip the fruit over and cook for a further 2 minutes until the fruit and nuts are golden.

Separately, cook the oats and remaining porridge ingredients in a small pot over low-medium heat, uncovered, for 5 minutes, stirring occasionally.

Serve oats in a bowl, with the topping of golden fruit, toasted nuts, coconut yoghurt, shredded coconut and the compote.

Drizzle with maple syrup or coconut sugar, if you like.

TIP: Experiment with different grains like semolina, quinoa or millet; dried fruit like cranberries, figs or apricots; and toasted seeds like hemp, sesame, sunflower and pepitas (hulled pumpkin seeds).

Use seasonal fruits, but always ensure they are cooked, to support Agni. In summer, reduce or remove the spices and serve with chopped mint and a dollop of coconut yoghurt.

Zesty rhubarb + ginger compote

A lovely accompaniment to breakfast dishes, like porridge and crispy crepes/pancakes. Rhubarb is an excellent source of vitamins, calcium and fibre that support bone and cardiovascular health. Naturally sweetened with antioxidant-rich red grape juice, this recipe pairs sweetness with tartness to create a zesty yet balanced compote.

1 teaspoon coconut oil

⅛ teaspoon cardamom seeds

1 x 2.5 cm (1 in) piece of fresh ginger, grated

½ teaspoon lemon rind

1 bunch (around 300 g) of fresh rhubarb stalks, roughly chopped

½ teaspoon ground cinnamon

pinch of sea salt

juice of half a lemon

⅓ cup (158 ml/2 ⅔ fl oz) red grape juice or ⅓ cup (158 ml/2 ⅔ fl oz) filtered water plus 1 teaspoon maple syrup

Up to 1 tablespoon jaggery or coconut sugar (optional)

Heat the oil in a small saucepan.

Add the cardamom seeds and fry for 1 minute until fragrant.

Add the grated ginger and lemon rind, and fry for 1 minute.

Add the rhubarb, cinnamon, salt, lemon juice and grape juice and simmer, covered, for 5-10 minutes, or until the rhubarb has broken down into a jam-like consistency.

Taste test and add jaggery or coconut sugar if necessary.

All-day crispy crepes (savoury)

Known as chillas or pudlas, these super simple 'chickpea crepes' or 'eggless pancakes' are absolutely delicious, super versatile and can be whipped together in minutes. They are gluten free and a great source of protein and fibre. Also delicious served with Stewed beans (page 152).

Makes 2

Base

½ cup (60 g / 2 ¼ oz) finely shredded seasonal vegetables (carrot, zucchini [courgette], cabbage, spring onion [scallion], leek, greens etc.)

1 cup (120 g/4½ oz) besan (chickpea flour)

¼ teaspoon ground cumin

¼ teaspoon ground turmeric

pinch of smoked paprika (optional)

pinch of sea salt, to taste

pinch of black pepper

pinch of asafoetida (hing) (optional – imparts a garlic flavour)

¾ cup (175 ml/6 fl oz) filtered water

1 teaspoon melted coconut oil or ghee

To serve

almond feta

fresh herbs

lemon juice

handful of chopped tomatoes

Wild pesto (page 161)

Ensure your chosen vegetables are finely shredded, chopped or grated to blend in well with the batter.

To make the crepes, put the flour, spices and salt in a mixing bowl and slowly add the water, whisking to make a smooth batter that you can pour with a ladle. You may need to add more water to reach this consistency.

Add the vegetables and fresh herbs to the batter and stir to combine well.

Using a non-stick pan, heat ½ teaspoon of the coconut oil or ghee over medium–high heat. Once the pan is hot (test by sprinkling in a drop of water, which will sizzle when the pan is at the right temperature), pour in half the batter and spread evenly.

Lower the heat a little and wait until bubbles cover the whole surface of the crepe (about 4–6 minutes). Drizzle with another ½ teaspoon of melted oil or ghee before flipping, then gently run a spatula over the crepe to make sure it is even.

Cook for a further 3–5 minutes, or until golden brown on both sides. Ensure the inside of the crepe has cooked through.

Repeat with the remaining batter.

Serve with toppings of your choice.

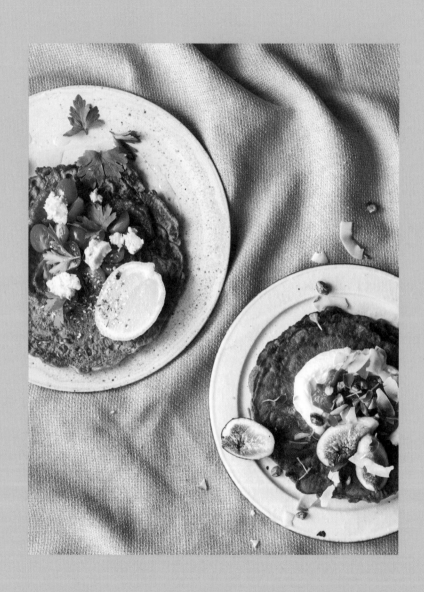

All-day crispy crepes (sweet)

If you're in the mood for something sweet and uplifting, combine your choice of seasonal fruit with protein-rich besan flour for a healthy pancake alternative.

Makes 2

Base

½ cup (60 g/2 ¼ oz) shredded /mashed seasonal fruit (banana, peach, apple, pear, fig etc.)

1 cup (120 g/4½ oz) besan (chickpea flour)

½ teaspoon ground cinnamon

pinch of ground cardamom

pinch of sea salt, to taste

1 tablespoon jaggery or coconut sugar

¾ cup (175 ml/6 fl oz) filtered water

2 teaspoons melted coconut oil or ghee

To serve

grilled fruit

toasted nuts and/or seeds

shredded coconut

coconut yoghurt

maple syrup

Zesty Rhubarb + Ginger Compote (page 146)

Ensure your chosen fruit is finely chopped, shredded, grated or mashed to blend in well with the batter.

To make the crepes, put the flour, cinnamon, cardamom, salt and jaggery, or coconut sugar, in a mixing bowl and slowly add the water, whisking to make a smooth batter that you can pour with a ladle. You may need to add more water to reach this consistency.

Add the fruit into the batter and stir to combine well.

Using a non-stick pan, heat ½ teaspoon of the oil, or ghee, over medium–high heat. Once the pan is hot (test by sprinkling in a drop of water, which will sizzle when the pan is at the right temperature), pour in half the batter and spread evenly.

Lower the heat a little and wait until bubbles cover the whole surface of the crepe (about 3–5 minutes). Drizzle with another ½ teaspoon of melted oil, or ghee, before flipping, then gently run a spatula over the crepe to make sure it is even.

Cook for a further 3–5 minutes, or until golden brown on both sides. Ensure the inside of the crepe has cooked through.

Repeat with the remaining batter.

Serve with toppings of your choice.

> TIP: Adjust the amount of water to suit your taste and the strength of your Agni (for those with low Agni, add more water for a lighter crepe; for those with strong Agni, you can use less water and enjoy as more of a pancake style).

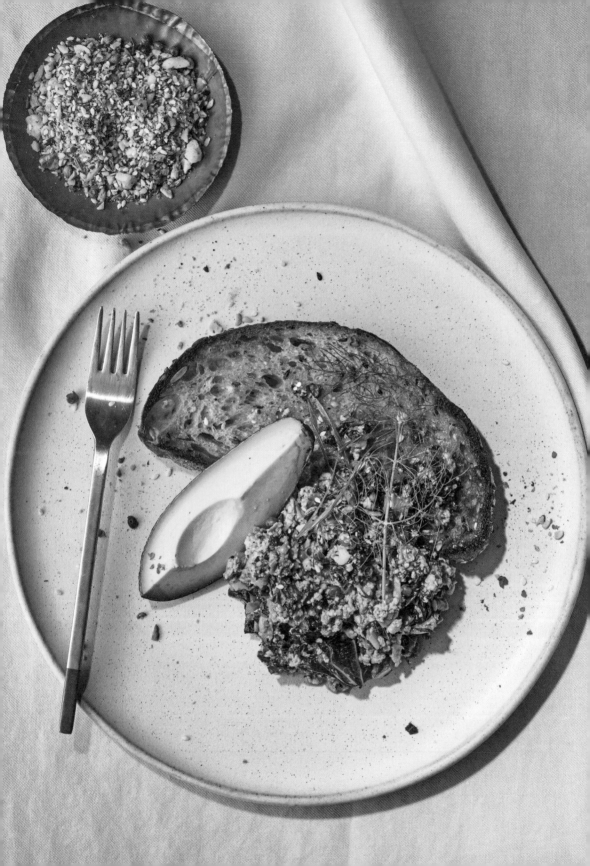

Spicy scrambled tofu

A wholesome, plant-based alternative to scrambled eggs made from creamy silken tofu, which is packed full of essential nutrients.

Serves 2

1 tablespoon coconut oil or ghee

¼ teaspoon cumin seeds (optional)

5 cm (2 in) piece of leek or half a brown onion

1 spring onion (scallion) stem

handful of baby spinach or 2 English spinach or silverbeet (chard) leaves

1 tablespoon fenugreek leaves (optional)

1 packet of silken tofu (300 g/10½ oz)

1 tablespoon coconut aminos (optional – imparts a sweet and salty depth)

¼ teaspoon ground cumin

¼ teaspoon ground turmeric

pinch of smoked paprika

pinch of asafoetida (hing)

½ teaspoon sea salt or black salt that contains sulphur (imparts the taste of egg)

pinch of black pepper

1 tablespoon nutritional yeast (optional – imparts a cheesy flavour)

1 tablespoon fresh herbs (dill, coriander [cilantro] and parsley work best)

To serve

toast

avocado

Toasted masala seed & nut churna (see page 170) (optional)

Heat the oil, or ghee, in a cast-iron pan over medium heat. Fry off the cumin seeds for 1 minute, if using. Add the leek/onion/scallions and cook until golden.

Add the spinach leaves and fenugreek leaves, if using, and cook until lightly sautéed.

Mash the tofu in a bowl with the back of a fork or simply break it up with your hands as you add it to the pan; it should be a crumbly/scrambled consistency.

Layer with coconut aminos, if using, and all of the remaining spices/seasoning and yeast, if using, and cook on medium heat for 5 minutes, stirring occasionally so that all of the tofu has been seasoned.

Add the fresh herbs and cook for 1 minute over high heat to give the tofu some body.

Serve with toast, avocado and toasted masala seed and nut churna.

TIP: You can add vegetables like mushrooms, broad beans, asparagus etc. to this dish; simply add them to the frying pan after the leek/onion/scallions and cook for a few minutes to soften, then add remaining ingredients. In summer, reduce or remove the spices (especially the smoked paprika) and serve with fresh chopped herbs and a squeeze of lemon.

Stewed beans

This dish is ideal in the wintertime when Agni is at its strongest and we require more fuel for our day. Also delicious paired with All-day crispy crepes (see page 147) or with rice and naan (see page 168).

Serves 2

1 cup (200 g/7 oz) dried black-eyed beans, washed and soaked overnight

2 cups (500 ml/17 fl oz) filtered water, plus more for soaking beans

½ teaspoon ground turmeric

½ teaspoon ground cumin

1 teaspoon sea salt

1 tablespoon ghee or coconut oil

pinch of cumin seeds

pinch of ajwain seeds or dried oregano (optional)

1 small brown onion, leek or spring onion (scallion), finely chopped

3 tomatoes, finely chopped

pinch of smoked paprika

pinch of asafoetida (hing)

pinch of black pepper

½ teaspoon jaggery or coconut sugar

1 tablespoon nutritional yeast (optional)

handful of chopped fresh herbs (coriander [cilantro], parsley, dill etc.)

To serve

Sweet potato rosti (see page 154)

parsley

almond feta

chilli flakes

Preparing the beans

Wash and soak black-eyed beans overnight in filtered water with a pinch of salt.

Rinse beans before use, discard bean shells, then add them to a large pot with 2 cups (500 ml/ 17 fl oz) filtered water, turmeric, ground cumin and ½ teaspoon of the sea salt. Cover and simmer on low heat.

To make the sauce

Melt the oil, or ghee, in a saucepan over medium heat. Add the cumin and ajwain seeds or dried oregano and fry for 1 minute. Add the onion/leek/ spring onion and fry until golden.

Add the chopped tomatoes, smoked paprika, hing, the remaining salt and the pepper. Cover and simmer on low heat for up to 20 minutes, stirring occasionally, until the tomatoes break down and the spices are infused, making a nice saucy consistency.

Add the sauce and jaggery, or coconut sugar, to the pot of beans and cook, uncovered, for a further 20 minutes, or until the beans are soft and the sauce has thickened.

Top with nutritional yeast for a cheesy flavour and serve with the sweet potato rosti. Sprinkle the feta, chilli flakes and any remaining fresh herbs on top.

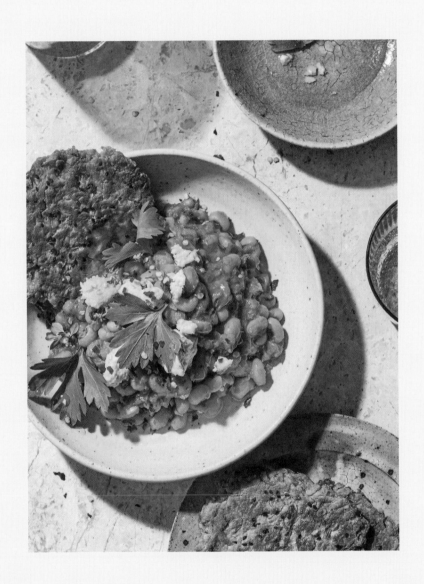

Sweet potato rosti

This is a lovely, earthy, grounding alternative to using bread or toast to accompany dishes but can also stand alone as a light breakfast, snack, simple dinner or as a delicious burger patty. Sweet potatoes possess the Earth element, as they are a root vegetable, which helps to ground Vata or flighty energy. They are packed full of essential vitamins and nutrients, help to cleanse and detoxify the gut and, despite being naturally sweet, they help to stabilise blood sugar levels, making this a perfect indulgence for those who enjoy a light, sweet, gluten-free meal.

Makes 6 patties

1 large sweet potato, grated (3 cups)

1 x 5 cm (2 in) piece of ginger, finely chopped (optional)

1 teaspoon grated lemon rind (optional)

½ cup finely chopped fresh herbs (dill, coriander [cilantro], parsley, spring onion [scallion] etc.)

1 cup (125 g/4½ oz) besan (chickpea flour) or 1 cup (125 g/4½ oz) buckwheat flour

1 teaspoon garam masala or curry powder

¼ teaspoon black cumin (nigella) seeds (optional)

pinch of salt, to taste

pinch of black pepper

½ teaspoon baking powder

1 tablespoon coconut oil or ghee

To serve
almond feta
chilli flakes
fresh herbs
Stewed beans (see page 152)

TIP: These are also great as a simple dinner paired with avocado, tahini, hummus, lemon and fresh greens.

Add the grated sweet potato to a large mixing bowl, along with the ginger, lemon rind and chopped herbs.

Mix the dried ingredients in a separate bowl, combining them well, then add them to the wet ingredients.

Using your hands, combine the wet and dry ingredients into a sticky batter, massaging the sweet potato to release its juices, and kneading the mix to bind it.

Divide the mixture into 6 balls and set aside.

Using a non-stick pan, heat the oil, or ghee, over medium-high heat. Once the pan is hot (test by sprinkling in a drop of water, which will sizzle when the pan is at the right temperature), place each ball individually in the pan and flatten it with the back of a spatula, making sure it is flattened quite thin. The size of the pan will determine how many fritters you can fit, but leave at least 2 cm (¾ in) between each.

Lower the heat a little and allow the fritters to cook thoroughly for 3-5 minutes before flipping them and cooking for a further 3-5 minutes. Once golden, check the inside is cooked through, then repeat the process with the remaining batter.

Serve with stewed beans and sprinkle feta, fresh herbs and chilli flakes on top.

TIP: This recipe also works well with cooked/baked sweet potato if you have some left over from another dish; simply mash it (instead of grating) and form patties with the batter.

In summer, this is a perfect, light dish, served with fresh chopped herbs or wild pesto and a squeeze of lemon.

Kitchari

An absolute staple in the Ayurvedic diet, Kitchari is a one-pot dish that is as quick and easy to prepare as it is to digest. As Kitchari has a balancing effect on all three Doshas, it has been used for thousands of years to support cleansing, detoxification, fasting and recovery. Kitchari is highly adaptable and this version can be made solely from dried ingredients, which means you can always create a meal even when the fridge is empty!

Serves 2

1 tablespoon coconut oil or ghee

¼ teaspoon black mustard seeds

¼ teaspoon cumin seeds

¼ teaspoon coriander (cilantro) seeds (optional)

¼ teaspoon ajwain seeds (optional)

1 cup (250 g/9 oz) split red lentils

½ cup (100 g/4½ oz) white basmati rice

1 teaspoon ground turmeric

1 teaspoon ground ginger

2–4 teaspoons garam masala or curry powder (to taste)

up to ½ teaspoon of salt, to taste

pinch of black pepper

pinch of asafoetida (hing) (optional)

6 cups (1.5 litres/51 fl oz) filtered or boiling water

To serve

fresh chopped coriander (cilantro)

Toasted masala seed & nut churna (see page 170)

Heat the oil, or ghee, in a heavy-bottomed pot.

Once the oil is hot, add the black mustard seeds and wait for them to pop – releasing their medicinal essential oils.

Turn down the heat and add the remaining seeds, then cook for
1 minute, being very careful not to burn them!

Add the washed lentils and rice to the pot, dust with the remaining spices and seasoning, and fry them all off for 2 minutes over medium heat, until the lentils are coated and the spices are aromatic.

Add either filtered or boiling water to the pot, bring to the boil, then simmer on a low heat, covered, for 30 minutes, stirring occasionally. The lentils should have dissolved into a saucy paste that binds the water to give it a creamy texture. This means the kitchari is ready!

Serve with coriander and toasted masala seed & nut churna.

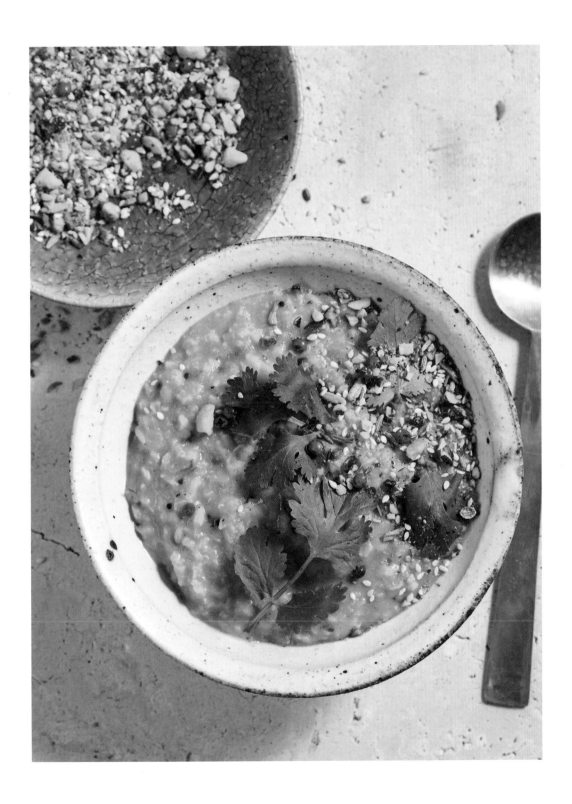

Fried seasonal greens

Green vegetables are an essential source of vitamins and antioxidants but can be difficult to digest on their own, which is why Ayurveda recommends cooking them with unctuous oils and spices to stimulate Agni and make their nutrients more bioavailable (easy to digest and absorb). This is a lovely dish to accompany other meals or as a standalone if you're in the mood for something light and nutritious.

Serves 1

1 teaspoon coconut oil or ghee

1 handful of seasonal greens (asparagus, green beans, broccolini, brussels sprouts, okra, silverbeet (chard), English spinach etc.)

1 teaspoon apple cider vinegar (optional)

1 teaspoon coconut aminos (optional)

¼ teaspoon ground fenugreek

¼ teaspoon ground cumin

pinch of asafoetida (hing) (optional)

pinch of sea salt

pinch of black pepper

To serve

fresh lemon

Toasted masala seed & nut Churna (see page 170)

Heat the oil, or ghee, in a cast-iron pan over medium heat.

Fry the greens for 2 minutes, then drizzle with the apple cider vinegar and coconut aminos, and dust with spices and seasoning. Cook for another 2 minutes, or until soft and golden.

Serve with a squeeze of lemon and a sprinkle of spice churna.

TIP: play around with your choice of spices

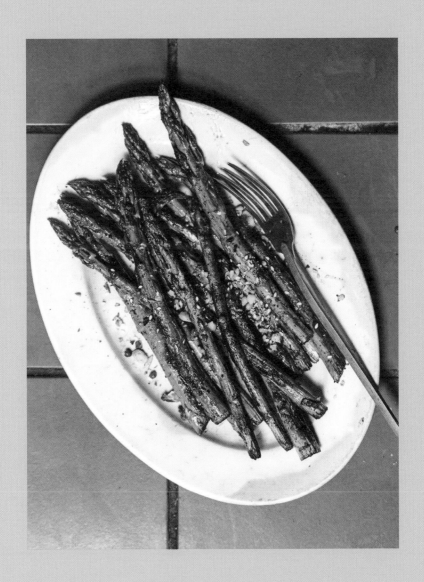

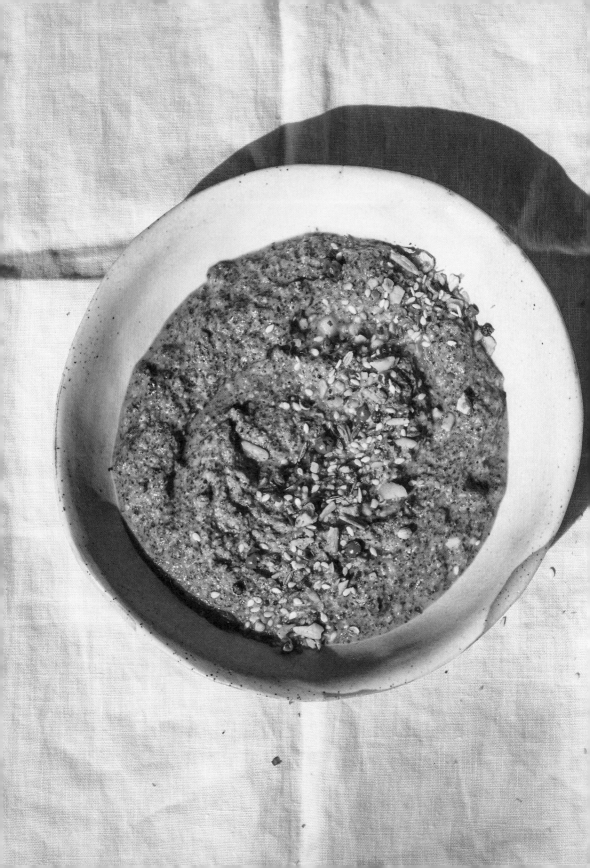

Wild pesto

There are no rules when it comes to crafting this delicious wild pesto! Grab whatever greens you have in your garden or fridge, or that you have foraged from around your neighbourhood, and whip them together with zesty lemon, tangy vinegar, unctuous oils and some spices, and voila! This is a nutrient-rich accompaniment that goes with pretty much anything under the sun. The greens help to 'put out the fire', or pacify Pitta (Fire element), meaning they are calming, soothing and help to detoxify the body and support the liver. They are also great for your skin. Shine from the inside out!

¼ teaspoon ajwain, cumin or coriander (cilantro) seeds, or a mix (optional)

½ cup pepitas (hulled pumpkin seeds)

1 large bunch of fresh greens (roughly 2 large handfuls) (dandelion/collard/ mustard greens, rocket [arugula], radicchio, lettuce, watercress, sorrel, tulsi 'holy basil', coriander [cilantro], basil, parsley, dill, mint etc.)

¼ teaspoon lemon rind

juice of half a lemon

pinch of sea salt, or more, to taste

pinch of black pepper

pinch of chilli flakes (optional)

1–2 tablespoons nutritional yeast (optional)

60 ml (4 fl oz) olive oil or avocado oil, plus 1 tablespoon olive oil for storing

1 tablespoon apple cider vinegar

Dry fry the seeds and pepitas in a cast-iron pan over low–medium heat. They burn easily, so keep them moving and remove them from the heat when they start to crackle.

If you want to do this the traditional way, finely chop all your greens, add them with the remaining ingredients to a large mortar and pestle, and massage until soft.

If you want to fast-track this process, whip them all together in a food processor.

Transfer the pesto to a clean jar and top with an extra tablespoon of olive oil to prevent mould from setting in. Store in the fridge.

Seasonal vegetable pie

A decadent pie loaded with nutritious vegetables and rich in fibre that can be made gluten-free. A mixture of mashed potato and barley is used to bind all of the ingredients together, meaning that this dish has the body to be baked naked or with pastry. There are a few stages involved in making this pie, so give yourself plenty of time and have patience. Perfect for occasions where you may like to offer something substantial and heart-warming.

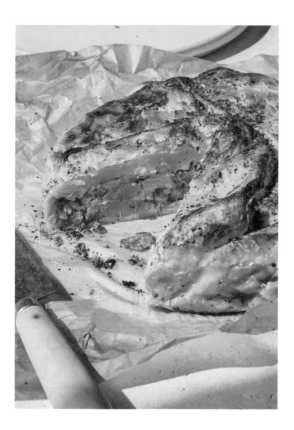

Baked vegetables

This is a guide; you can use a selection of seasonal vegetables suited to your needs.

2 tablespoons melted coconut oil or ghee

1 small white potato

1 small sweet potato

1 small beetroot (beet)

1 carrot

1 leek

¼ cauliflower

2 tomatoes

½ teaspoon ground turmeric

1 tablespoon garam masala or curry powder

1 teaspoon sea salt

pinch of black pepper

Grains

¼ cup (55 g/2 oz) barley

¾ cup (125 ml/6 fl oz) filtered water

1 stock cube or ¼ teaspoon ground cumin plus ¼ teaspoon ground turmeric and a pinch of salt to taste

TIP: Feel free to use any variations of seasonal vegetables in this mix and play around with the spices to suit your palate. In summer, reduce the amount of spices and serve at room temperature with a side salad.

Mashed potatoes

2 small white potatoes, cubed

2 cups (500 ml/17 fl oz) water

1 stock cube

½ cup (125 ml/ 4 fl oz) nut milk

1 tablespoon ghee or olive oil

¼ teaspoon sea salt

pinch of black pepper

1–2 tablespoons nutritional yeast
(optional)

Fresh

handful of chopped English spinach

handful of fresh parsley

Other

1 sheet of good quality puff pastry,
27 cm x 27 cm (10¾ in x 10¾ in)
(optional)

½ cup (75 g/2¾ oz) feta – almond/
dairy (optional)

1 teaspoon toasted masala seed
+ nut churna (see page 170),
to garnish top (optional)

To serve

fresh green side salad (optional)

Wild pesto (see page 161) (optional)

Wash and cube vegetables of your choice for baking, then add them to a mixing bowl with the melted oil, or ghee, and spices. Mix through and place on a baking tray. Bake at 180°C (350°F) for 45–60 minutes, or until cooked and golden, but not overly soft as they will continue to cook when the pie is baked.

Wash the barley thoroughly. In a small saucepan, bring the barley to the boil in the filtered water with the stock or seasoning, then cover and simmer over a low heat for 20 minutes; turn off the heat and allow to sit for 10 minutes, covered.

Boil the potatoes in the water with the stock cube for 15 minutes, covered, then drain, mash with the nut milk, oil, salt and pepper and nutritional yeast, if using.

Once all of the above ingredients are ready, in a large mixing bowl add the vegetables, barley, mashed potato, fresh spinach and parsley. Combine well and allow to cool in the fridge for 15–30 minutes.

Line a 20 cm × 20 cm (7 in × 7 in) baking tray or pie dish with baking paper and, if using, lay your pastry out, centring it so that its edges fall evenly over the sides of the dish or tray (the pastry will be folded back over the filling) and add your filling.

Top with the feta, if using, then fold the edges of the pastry over, if using, to encase the filling, and lightly sprinkle with spice churna. Bake for 15 minutes on 200°C (400°F), then lower the heat to 180°C (350°F) and cook until golden, about 15–30 minutes.

Serve with a side salad and wild pesto, if including

Seasonal mixed vegetable curry

This is a great one-pot dish to have if you're feeling a little 'under the weather' or just to get your daily dose of nature's medicine!

Serves 2

1 tablespoon coconut oil or ghee

⅛ teaspoon black mustard seeds

⅛ teaspoon cumin seeds

⅛ teaspoon coriander (cilantro) seeds

1 leek, finely chopped

1 x 5 cm (2 in) piece of ginger, finely chopped or grated

3 medium tomatoes, diced

½ teaspoon ground turmeric

2–4 teaspoons garam masala or curry powder (to taste)

½ teaspoon sea salt

pinch of black pepper

pinch of asafoetida (hing) (optional – imparts garlic flavour)

2 cups (250 ml/8½ fl oz) filtered water

4 cups seasonal vegetables, cubed (keep root vegetables, softer vegetables and greens separate)

To serve

fresh coriander (cilantro)

grain of choice: rice, quinoa, barley etc.

Homemade naan bread (see page 168)

Tangy coconut raita (see page 169)

Heat the oil, or ghee, in a heavy-bottomed pot over medium heat. Once the oil is hot, add the black mustard seeds and wait for them to pop. Turn down the heat and add the remaining seeds, then cook for 1 minute, being very careful not to burn them!

Fry off the leek and ginger until golden.

Add the diced tomatoes with the ground spices and seasoning, and cook, covered, for around 10 minutes, until the tomatoes have broken down.

Add the water and allow it to bind with the tomatoes, creating a saucy consistency, then cook, uncovered, for a further 10 minutes.

Begin to add the seasonal vegetables to the pot in stages, based on their cooking time. Root vegetables will go in first and need up to 20 minutes to cook, softer vegetables go in next for an additional 10 minutes, and any greens go in last for about 5 minutes. Use your intuition to guide you and keep checking the textures. Keep the lid on while cooking so the sauce doesn't evaporate.

Once all the vegetables have softened and the sauce has thickened, your curry is ready!

Serve on its own or with a grain, coriander, naan, and/or raita.

Saag aloo (spinach + potato) curry

Rich in essential vitamins, this powerhouse
dish will make you glow from the inside out.

Serves 2

1 tablespoon coconut oil or ghee

¼ teaspoon fenugreek seeds

¼ teaspoon cumin seeds

¼ teaspoon coriander
(cilantro) seeds

1 leek, finely chopped

1 x 5 cm (2 in) piece of ginger,
finely chopped

3 medium tomatoes, diced
(optional)

½ teaspoon ground coriander
(cilantro)

2–4 teaspoons garam masala
or curry powder (to taste)

pinch of asafoetida (hing)

½ teaspoon sea salt

pinch of black pepper

2 cups (250 ml/8½ fl oz) filtered
water

3 medium potatoes (of your
choice), washed and cubed

1 tablespoon dried fenugreek
leaves or curry leaves
(optional)

4 cups of English spinach,
silverbeet (chard) or baby
spinach, finely chopped

1 handful of fresh coriander
(cilantro) leaves and stems,
finely chopped

½ cup (125 ml) coconut milk
or coconut cream (optional)

To serve

squeeze of lemon

fresh coriander (cilantro)

grain of choice: rice, quinoa, barley etc.

Homemade naan bread(see page 168)

Tangy coconut raita (see page 169)

Heat the oil, or ghee, in a heavy-bottomed pot over
medium heat. Once the oil is hot, fry the seeds for
about 1 minute, being very careful not to burn them!

Fry off the leek and ginger until golden.

Add the diced tomatoes with the ground spices
and seasoning, and simmer, covered, for around 10
minutes, until the tomatoes have broken down.

Add the water and allow it to bind with the tomatoes,
creating a saucy consistency, then cook over medium
heat, uncovered, for a further 10 minutes.

Add the cubed potatoes and cook for 15–20 minutes
with the lid on.

Once they are almost soft, add the fenugreek/curry
leaves, spinach, coriander stems. Stir through and
cook, covered, stirring occasionally, until the greens
have wilted and softened. They should bind with the
sauce to form a creamy consistency. This could take
up to 45 minutes.

Five minutes before serving, add the coconut milk or
cream, if using.

Serve with lemon, fresh coriander, rice, naan and/
or raita.

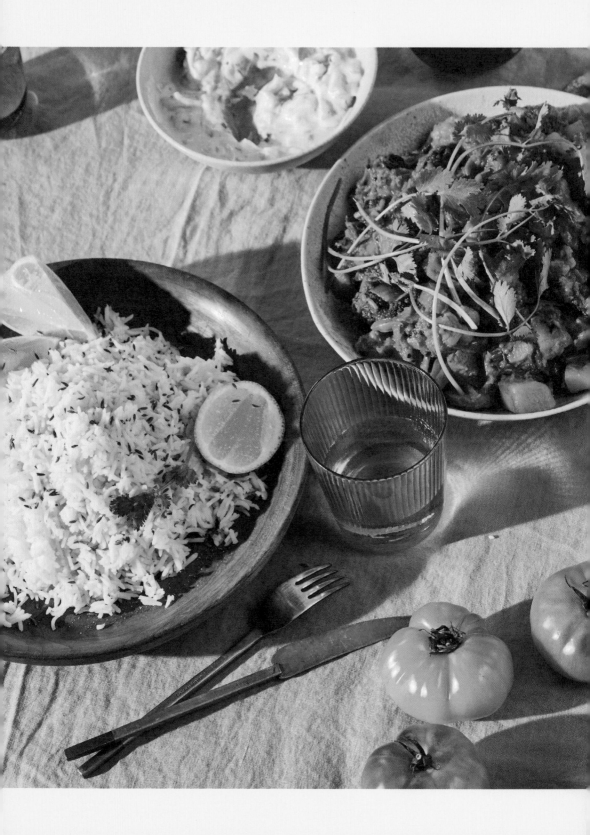

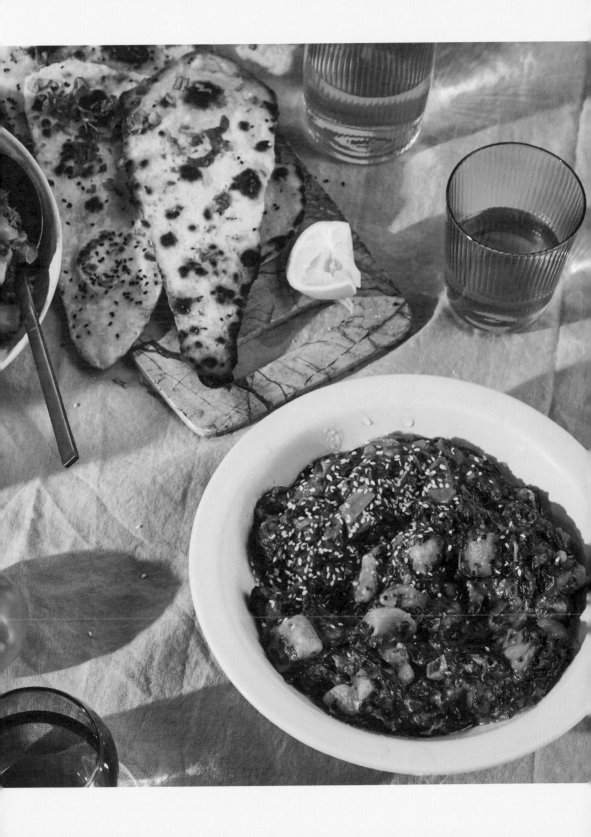

Homemade naan bread

A quick and easy traditional homemade naan bread that can be kept simple or jazzed up with spices and seasonings of your choice. The best part about this recipe is that you don't need to let it rest before cooking, so it can be whipped up in minutes to accompany your favourite dishes.

Makes 4 naan breads

1 cup (150 g/5½ oz) plain flour (all-purpose)

½ cup (125 g/4½ oz) yoghurt of your choice (ensure that it is unflavoured and unsweetened)

1 tablespoon apple cider vinegar

1 teaspoon baking powder

¼ teaspoon sea salt

¼ teaspoon black cumin (nigella) seeds (optional)

2 tablespoons ghee or coconut oil, melted

handful of fresh chopped parsley (optional)

½ lemon (optional)

Using your hands, combine the flour, yoghurt, vinegar, baking powder and salt together well in a large mixing bowl. The batter will be quite sticky at first; add more flour if necessary, until you can work it into a ball. You don't need to knead it overly or let it rest.

Remove it from the bowl and place it on a floured surface. Cut the ball into quarters.

Using a rolling pin, flatten one quarter into an oval shape and sprinkle with a few nigella seeds on the top, if using.

Heat a non-stick pan or cast-iron skillet over medium–high heat. Once it's hot, add a teaspoon of oil, or ghee, and cook one portion of naan until it bubbles; about 2 minutes. Top it with another teaspoon of melted oil, flip it and cook for a further 1–2 minutes.

Repeat with the remaining portions of dough.

Serve the naan with a squeeze of lemon juice and chopped parsley, if using.

TIP: Roll out each quarter individually while one naan is cooking, to prevent the naan from sticking to the rolling surface. The naan can be reheated in the oven or toaster. The dough can be kept in the fridge for 3 days; when ready to cook, simply flour your surface, roll out the naan and cook as desired.

Tangy coconut raita

Yoghurt is a cornerstone of many Ayurvedic meals and is served alongside spicy curries to temper the heat. Raita is a traditional yoghurt-based sauce, enriched with the subtle cooling properties of cucumber and mint, with the addition of some tangy and spicy flavours that are combined to create balance. It's so simple to make and elevates all well-seasoned dishes. Make sure your yoghurt is unsweetened and unflavoured.

1 cup (250 ml/8½ fl oz) plain coconut yoghurt

⅓ cup peeled and grated cucumber (cucumber skin is notoriously difficult to digest)

1 tablespoon spring onion (scallion), finely chopped

1 tablespoon fresh mint, finely chopped

pinch of cayenne pepper or smoked paprika (optional)

¼ teaspoon ground cumin

up to 1 tablespoon apple cider vinegar (optional)

pinch of sea salt, to taste

filtered water, as desired

Simply whisk all of the ingredients together, apart from the salt and water, in a mixing bowl, then slowly add salt and water to reach your desired taste and consistency.

Enjoy immediately or store in a jar in the fridge.

Toasted masala seed + nut churna

Much like dukkah or za'atar, this is a blend of traditional Ayurvedic spices accompanied by a variety of nutrient-rich toasted nuts and seeds to create a perfectly balanced, earthy garnish packed full of iron, calcium and zinc. You can switch out the pistachios and macadamias for any nuts of your choice. You can also add local spices to the mix, such as pepperleaf, wattleseed, lemon myrtle etc.

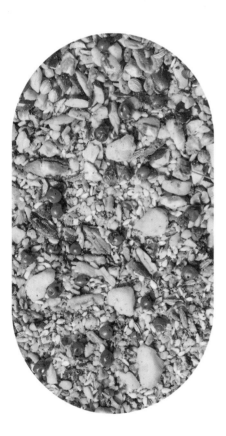

¼ cup (35 g/1¼ oz) pistachios

¼ cup (40 g/1½ oz) macadamias

¼ cup (30 g/1 oz) pepitas (hulled pumpkin seeds)

¼ cup (30 g/1 oz) sunflower seeds

1 teaspoon pink peppercorns

1 teaspoon cumin seeds

1 teaspoon coriander (cilantro) seeds

1 teaspoon fennel seeds

¼ cup (40 g/1½ oz) white sesame seeds

½ teaspoon ground turmeric

pinch of salt, to taste

Finely chop, crush or blend the pistachios, macadamias, pepitas and sunflower seeds individually so they are no larger than a peppercorn.

Heat a cast-iron pan over medium heat, then add the peppercorns, cumin, coriander and fennel seeds, and dry fry for 1 minute.

Add all of the remaining ingredients and toast for another 2–3 minutes or until the nuts are golden.

Separate half of the mixture and grind it in a mortar and pestle, or food processor, so that you have a nice blend of textures between the ground and whole ingredients. (optional)

Store in an airtight container.

One of the fundamental aspects of the Ayurvedic diet is consuming foods that have undergone the application of heat. **Pakti** is a Sanskrit term that shares a few meanings, such as 'cooked', 'digestion' and 'dignity'. By cooking your meals, you are actually assisting with the first stage of digestion by making your food bioavailable, meaning that the nutrients are much more accessible when they enter the body. This is far removed from the recent trend of the raw food diet; although raw veggies 'may' contain more vitamins and nutrients, they can be harder or even impossible for our bodies to metabolise. Visualise a raw piece of carrot entering our soft and supple digestive tract, which has to try and break down such a rigid material. The rule is, if you can't dissolve the food between the tongue and roof of the mouth, chances are your gut won't be able to either. Now imagine that the carrot has been sautéed or softened through any form of cooking – the cellular structure has become much softer and can be penetrated by our enzymes and the gut. Even when raw food has been blended or juiced, the cellular structure still remains intact and can be challenging for digestion. Ayurveda recommends that at least 80 per cent of your diet should be cooked, with room for light salads and fruit based on your constitution and the seasons.

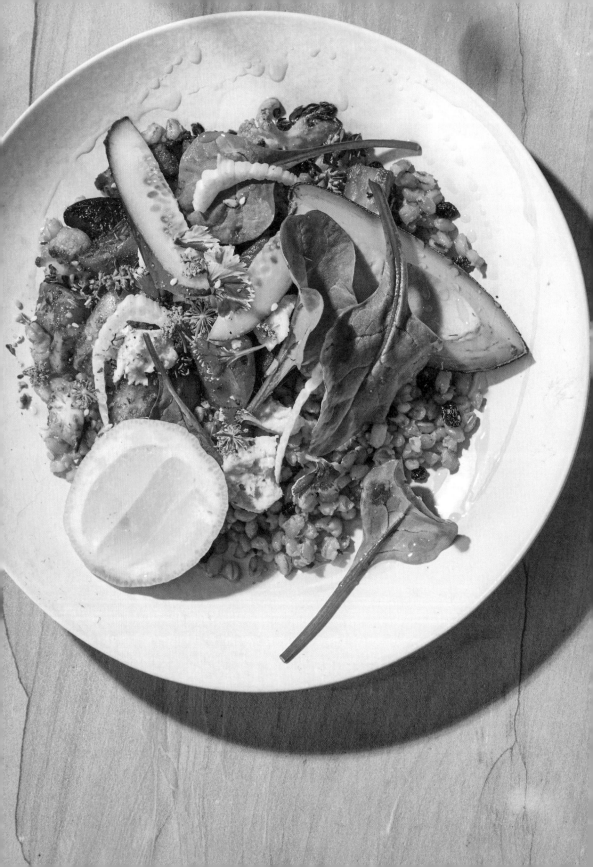

Warm pakti bowl

Think of this dish as a cooked, warm salad you can customise to suit your needs and whip together based on what you have on hand. This recipe is just one of the hundreds of ways you can craft and create your own pakti bowls. The guideline is: one-third grains, one-third cooked vegetables and one-third salad, topped with unctuous oils to support Agni.

Serves 2

Baked vegetables

1 small sweet potato

1 small beetroot (beet)

1 leek

1 tablespoon melted coconut oil or ghee

½ teaspoon ground turmeric

up to 1 tablespoon garam masala or curry powder

pinch of sea salt

pinch of black pepper

Grains

½ cup (110 g/4 oz) barley, or grain of your choice

1 cup (250 ml/8½ fl oz) filtered water

1 stock cube or ¼ teaspoon ground cumin plus ¼ teaspoon ground turmeric and ¼ teaspoon salt

1 teaspoon currants (optional)

To serve

squeeze of lemon

1 tablespoon olive, hemp or avocado oil

1 tablespoon apple cider vinegar

handful of fresh salad greens

fresh herbs

cucumber, thinly sliced

fennel, thinly sliced

avocado

almond feta

Wash and cube vegetables of your choice for baking, then add them to a mixing bowl with the melted oil and spices. Mix through and place on a baking tray. Bake at 180°C (350°F) for 45–60 minutes, or until cooked through and golden.

Wash the barley (or your grain of choice) thoroughly. In a small saucepan, bring to the boil with the water, stock or seasoning and salt, then cover and simmer over a low heat for 20 minutes; turn off the heat and allow to sit for 10 minutes, covered.

Wash and prepare your fresh ingredients.

Once the baked vegetables are ready, layer your bowl with grains and root vegetables, with the fresh salad ingredients and herbs on the side. Dress with oil, lemon and vinegar, and serve with a sprinkle of feta and currants on top.

Spiced almond tahini bites

These soft, gooey bites are super quick to make with only a few, nutritious ingredients that increase energy and relieve nausea, pain and inflammation. There are two flavour options or you can experiment with making a mixed batch.

Makes 12

Base

¼ cup (60 ml/2 fl oz) hulled tahini

¼ cup (60 ml/2 oz) nut butter

¼ cup (60 ml/2 fl oz) maple syrup

1 teaspoon vanilla extract

2 cups ground almonds

pinch of salt

chopped pistachios/nuts, sesame seeds, coconut flakes, rose petals etc., for garnishing

Red velvet

1 tablespoon ground beetroot (beets)

½ teaspoon ground cinnamon

½ teaspoon ground ginger

½ teaspoon rose powder

pinch of ground cardamom

Golden chai

½ tablespoon ground turmeric

½ teaspoon ground cinnamon

½ teaspoon ground ginger

pinch of nutmeg

pinch of pepper

Preheat the oven to 170°C (340°F (convection) /150°C (300°F) (fan-forced). Line a baking tray with baking paper.

Start by making the base. Mix the tahini, nut butter, maple syrup and vanilla in a small mixing bowl. If the ingredients are solid, you can do this over a low heat in a small saucepan to soften and combine well.

In a mixing bowl, add the ground almonds and your choice of either red velvet or golden chai spices.

Pour the tahini mixture into the ground almonds (be sure to split it evenly if doing a mixed batch) and mix to combine into a rough dough.

Use an ice-cream scooper, tablespoon or your hands to form 12 balls out of the mixture.

Place them on the baking tray and flatten with the palm of your hand.

If decorating, add toppings of your choice and gently press them into the tops to secure.

Bake in the preheated oven for approximately 10 minutes. Switch off the heat and let them brown slightly in the hot oven for another 5 minutes before removing.

Cool on a wire rack for about half an hour; they will firm up during this time.

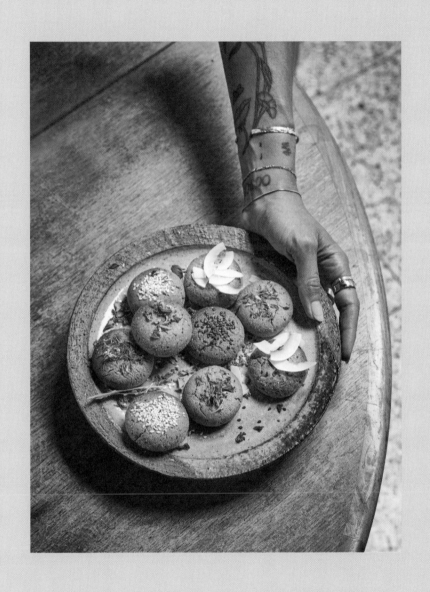

ELIXIRS

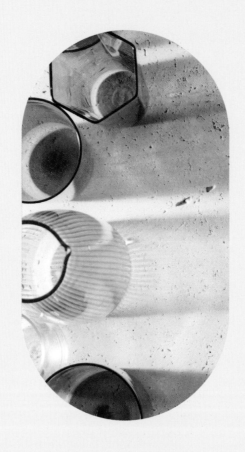

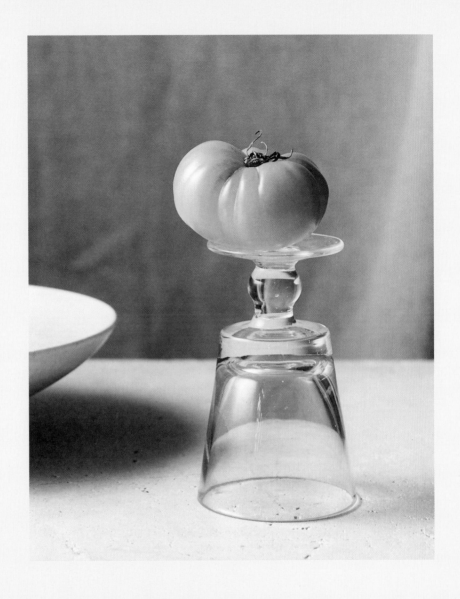

9

Elixirs of life

In a lifestyle that respects the elements of the natural world, the consumption of anything artificial is seen as taboo, so it's no surprise that Ayurveda leans away from any beverages outside of water, herbal tea and milk varieties.

Sodium, which is used to give fizz to soft drinks and soda water (club soda), is Vata aggravating (as it is largely made up of the Air element) and can deplete magnesium stores and weaken bones and teeth, even hair and nails, as they are all made from the same tissue. And this is not to mention the detrimental effects of the artificial colours, flavours and sugars found in soft drinks. Naturally sparkling mineral water is okay on occasion, but it is still prone to aggravate Vata if taken in excess.

When it comes to drinking water, there is a common misconception that we should carry an enormous bottle everywhere we go and constantly be knocking it back. Yes, hydration is absolutely essential for health, but consuming large quantities of water – especially when gulped down, cold or straight from the tap without filtration – can actually cause dehydration. How? We have a unique balance of acids, enzymes and pancreatic juices that live in the stomach, and by consuming excessive amounts of water we are drastically diluting them, which can cause great difficulty when it comes to breaking down our food. What should be a nectar of acidity needed for digestion becomes a stretched-out watery version of itself, which is far less effective – and detrimental to anyone suffering with low Agni. Excessive water consumption also flushes out and leeches away the essential nutrients, salts and minerals we need from water, lowering the body's store of salt and electrolytes and leaving us dehydrated. By drinking less and adding a tiny pinch of good quality salt to your water, you have a better chance of retaining minerals and staying hydrated while reducing the risk of dilution and dehydration.

Most of our water content should come from our food, believe it or not. When a grain of rice, or bean, has been soaked and boiled, it contains anywhere from 50–70 per cent water content, which provides an excellent source of hydration for the body. Same goes for fruit and vegetables, which are largely made up of water. By consuming a diet rich in fresh produce and cooked foods, you should be flooding your body with ample amounts of water, with the addition of herbal teas, sipping cups of water when thirsty and practising Ushapaan (see page 54). The quality of your water is also incredibly important. Tap water is laced with harmful chemicals used to sterilise the water, which can become damaging to your health. Old pipes used to transport water are also a melting pot for bacteria. It is essential to filter your water before drinking it or cooking with it to avoid the addition of unwanted toxins.

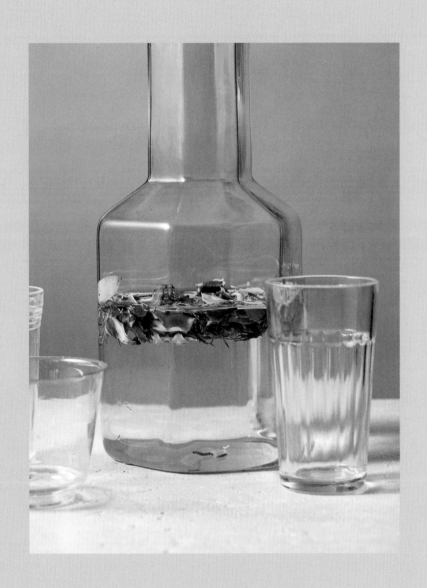

Medicinal teas

Medicinal teas work to subtly impart their healing vibrations on a daily basis, contributing to the overall practice of restoring health and wellbeing.

Infusing hot water with the magic of the plant kingdom is alchemy at its finest. Taking a herb, flower, leaf or root and making it medicine is a beautiful gift that Ayurveda cherishes, offering many healing recipes to suit your personal needs. By cultivating a relationship with this diverse array of healing elixirs you are one step closer to becoming your own healer.

No matter what the imbalance, Mother Nature has designed a plant to complement and soothe every condition and restore balance. There are plants to lift your mood, help you sleep, relieve you of anxiety and stress, support your liver and cleanse your blood, detoxify your system, aid digestion, soothe respiratory conditions, empower libido, clear skin conditions, improve your brainpower and enhance memory – whatever health ailments pop up, there is a plant to help navigate your way back to balance.

Start to cultivate a collection of these dried herbs, which you can experiment with as needed. They work well in combination with each other, so play around with the properties you need and the combination of flavour profiles that suits your taste.

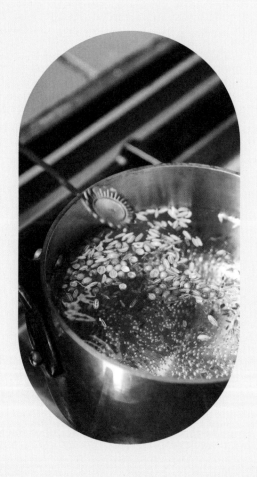

HERBAL TEAS AND INFUSIONS

Steep dried or fresh plants in boiling water for 10–20 minutes, then strain and sip. Alternatively, soak overnight and consume the tea throughout the day. Various suggestions are included below for a range of conditions.

Skin conditions:

o   CCF tea (see page 130)

o   Calendula (soothing and healing)

o   Neem powder or leaf (clears infections and irritations)

o   Turmeric and black pepper (cleanses impurities and clears infections, antibiotic)

o   Fenugreek (anti-ageing)

o   Manjistha (blood and skin cleansing)

Liver support:

o   Dandelion root (a strong diuretic that is useful in bladder conditions and UTIs, and to reduce swelling/inflammation)

o   Neem leaf

o   Turmeric

o   Black pepper

Hormone balancing:

o   Raspberry leaf

o   Mugwort

o   Motherwort

o   Sage

o   Shatavari

Sleep conditions:

o   Brahmi

o   Chamomile

o   Lavender

o   Licorice

o   Cardamom

o   Passionflower

Emotional support:

o   Rose petals/buds

o   Hibiscus

o   Sage

o   Tulsi

o   Lavender

Mental unrest (stress, anxiety, depression, mood swings):

o   Brahmi

o   Tulsi

o   Chamomile

o   Rose

o   Sage

o   Tagar/Valerian

o   Passionflower

Cognitive function (memory, alertness):

o   Brahmi

o   Tulsi

o   Gotu Kola

Iron supplement:

o   Nettle

o   Raspberry leaf

o   Dandelion

Pain relief:

o   Ginger (suits nausea, cramps, muscle and joint pain, inflammation)

o   Peppermint (headaches, migraines, excess heat, hot flushes)

o   Ajwain seeds (period pain, cramps, indigestion, bloating, gas)

o   Cinnamon (suits inflammation, aching bones and cramps)

Respiratory support:

o   Tulsi

o   Peppermint

o   Cinnamon

o   Ginger

o   Lemongrass

o   Licorice (especially useful in preventing asthma attacks)

TIP: Please be aware that if you are trying to conceive or are currently pregnant it is recommended that you seek advice from your health practitioner to discuss which teas are suitable for you.

LOVELY COMBINATIONS

Morning brew:
I love to start the day with 2 tablespoons of dandelion tea brewed in a French press as a chocolate-brown, caffeine-free, liver-cleansing coffee alternative. On certain mornings when I need a bit of a kickstart, I might add between 1 teaspoon and 1 tablespoon of organic ground coffee in the mix. They make for a dreamy partnership. You can add a pinch of cardamom powder to neutralise the effects of the caffeine.

Anti-inflammatory pain reliever and respiratory relief:
⅛ teaspoon each of ground turmeric, cinnamon, ginger and cardamom with a pinch of black pepper, steeped or boiled in a pot of boiling water.

As an option, you can add a squeeze of lemon and ½ teaspoon maple syrup or jaggery.

Nutrient blast and hormone stabiliser:
1 teaspoon each of dried nettle leaf, peppermint leaf, raspberry leaf, brahmi leaf, tulsi leaf and lemon myrtle leaf brewed in a pot of boiling water.

Sleepy tea:
1 teaspoon each of chamomile flowers, lavender tips, licorice root and valerian root brewed in a pot of boiling water.

Heart healer:
1 teaspoon each of rose petals/buds, hibiscus, lavendar, sage leaves and tulsi leaves brewed in a pot of boiling water.

Liver and skin cleanser:
½ teaspoon each of ground turmeric, cinnamon, manjistha and a pinch of black pepper in a pot of boiling water. Stir well.

DOSHA-BALANCING PLANTS/TEAS

Vata:
Ginger, cloves, cardamom, nutmeg, cinnamon, saffron, sage, star anise, licorice.

Pitta:
Mint, fennel, chamomile, coriander (cilantro), cardamom, saffron, fenugreek, brahmi, rose.

Kapha:
Turmeric, black pepper, ginger, fenugreek, cloves, brahmi, tulsi.

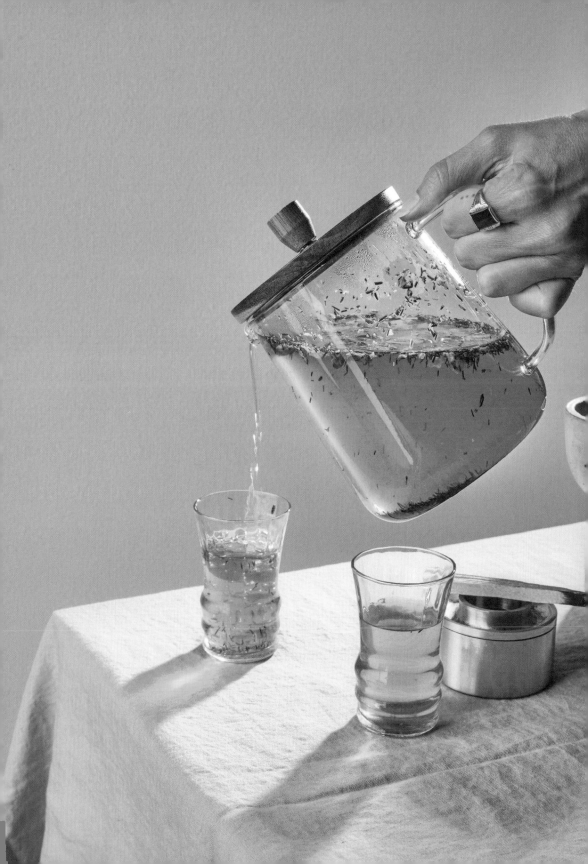

Milk-based elixirs

These wholesome milk-based tea blends have been crafted to flood the body with the healing powers of the plant kingdom while providing energy and satisfaction. Each recipe has variations for stimulation (sun milk) or unwinding (moon milk).

'Sun milks' are energy boosting and include ingredients that help to switch on and activate the body and mind so you can power through your day; they are best taken before midday. 'Moon milks' are soothing and comforting night-time elixirs that are known for their ability to inspire a deep night's sleep. In Ayurveda, warm milk consumed before bed is a common remedy for sleeplessness, anxiety and insomnia. Moon milk in its simplest form consists of plain warm milk but can be supercharged with the addition of calming herbs and spices such as turmeric, cinnamon, nutmeg, lavender, blue lotus, passionflower and cornflower – to name a few.

Crafting tips:

o Use your choice of milk, nut milk or try making your own!

o Experiment with your variation of milk and water to reach your desired consistency.

o Both coconut oil and ghee help with the absorption and transportation of vitamins and nutrients to the parts of the body that need them most.

o If you're in the mood for something sweet, try adding up to ½ teaspoon jaggery, coconut sugar or maple syrup per serve.

o For an extra creamy experience, use a handheld milk frother or whisk to add more body.

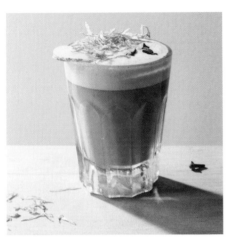
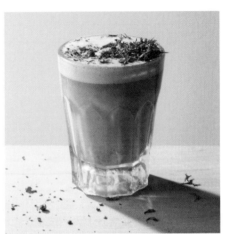
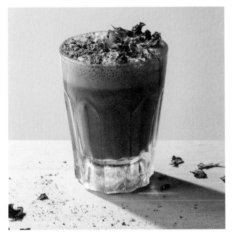
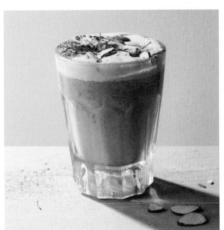

Vedic chai

Chai (Masala) is used as a preventative and curative of disease. Its nourishing mix of medicinal herbs and spices is known for its anti-inflammatory and antioxidant value.

Serves 1

1 cm (½ in) piece of ginger root, sliced or grated, or ¼ teaspoon ground ginger

¼ teaspoon ground cinnamon

seeds from 1 cracked cardamom pod or a pinch of ground cardamom

1 clove (optional)

pinch of black pepper

½ cup (125 ml/4 fl oz) water

1 teaspoon black tea leaves

½ cup (125 ml/4 fl oz) milk (of your choice)

drop of coconut oil or ghee (optional)

up to teaspoon sweetener of your choice (optional)

cinnamon, star anise, cloves, or orange peel, for garnishing

Bring ginger, spices and water to the boil in a small pot, covered.

Reduce the heat and add the tea leaves, and simmer, covered, for a further 2 minutes.

Add the milk and simmer on a low heat, uncovered, for a further 5 minutes.

Strain into a large mug with room for whisking. Then add sweetener and oil and stir or whisk until smooth and fluffy.

Dust with cinnamon powder or the garnish of your choice.

TIP: Sun milk – opt for black tea leaves that include a small amount of caffeine for an energy boost.

Moon milk – substitute black tea leaves with dandelion or rooibos tea for a caffeine-free alternative and add a pinch of nutmeg for a calming night-time elixir.

Golden milk

This elixir supports digestive health, boosts the immune system, soothes pain and inflammation, and contributes to overall health and longevity.

Serves 1

¼ teaspoon ground turmeric

¼ teaspoon ground ginger

¼ teaspoon ground cinnamon

pinch of ground nutmeg

pinch of vanilla bean powder
  or essence (optional)

pinch of black pepper

½ cup (125 ml/4 fl oz) water

½ cup (125 ml/4 fl oz) milk
  (of your choice)

drop of coconut oil or ghee
  (optional)

up to ½ teaspoon sweetener
  of your choice (optional)

cracked pepper, dried
  lavender, cornflower,
  passionflower or blue lotus,
  for garnishing

Bring spices and water to the boil in a small pot, covered.

Reduce the heat and add the milk, and simmer on low heat, uncovered, for a further 5 minutes.

Strain into a large mug with room for whisking. Then add sweetener and oil and stir or whisk until smooth and fluffy.

Dust with cracked pepper and dried flowers of your choice

TIP: Sun milk – don't include the nutmeg.

Moon milk – include the nutmeg and the dried flowers.

Dandelion rose cacao

Dandelion plants help to reduce water retention, oedema, high blood pressure, toxins and inflammation, while flooding the body with potent antioxidants. This drink is an antidote for depression, heartache or unresolved trauma.

Serves 1

1 teaspoon roasted dandelion root

½ cup (125 ml/4 fl oz) water

1-2 teaspoons cacao powder, to taste

1 teaspoon rosewater

pinch of rose powder (optional)

pinch of vanilla bean powder or essence (optional)

½ cup (125 ml/4 fl oz) milk of your choice

drop of coconut oil or ghee (optional)

up ½ to teaspoon sweetener of your choice

cacao powder and 3 rose petals, for garnishing

Bring dandelion, cacao, rose powder, vanilla and water to the boil in a small pot, covered.

Reduce the heat and add the milk, and simmer on low heat, uncovered, for a further 5 minutes.

Strain into a large mug with room for whisking. Then add sweetener and oil and stir or whisk until smooth and fluffy.

Garnish with rose petals.

Note: this recipe requires a sweetener to balance the bitterness of the cacao and dandelion.

TIP: Sun milk – cacao is quite stimulating, so this drink is best taken in the morning or before 12 pm. This elixir is a wonderful, energising replacement for coffee.

Moon milk – leave out the cacao and replace it with a pinch of nutmeg.

Ojas booster

This elixir can be used to restore energy after physical exertion, sex or emotional depletion. This is also a nurturing, anti-inflammatory elixir to soothe any type of inflammation as well as period pain while boosting the immune system.

Serves 1

1 Medjool date, deseeded and finely chopped

¼ teaspoon ground cinnamon

pinch of ground cardamom

pinch of ground nutmeg

pinch of vanilla bean powder or essence (optional)

1 strand of saffron

½ cup (125 ml/4 fl oz) water

½ cup (125 ml/4 fl oz) almond milk

drop of coconut oil or ghee (optional)

flaked almond, dried calendula, and/or saffron strands, for garnishing

Bring the chopped date, spices and water to the boil in a small pot, covered, for 5 minutes.

Reduce the heat and add the almond milk, and simmer on low heat, uncovered, for a further 5 minutes.

Pour into a large mug with room for whisking. Then add oil (if using) and stir, whisk or blend until smooth and the dates have broken down.

Dust with cinnamon, flowers, saffron and flaked almonds.

Note: this recipe does not require a sweetener due to the nature of the Medjool date.

TIP: Sun milk – leave out the nutmeg. Moon milk – include the nutmeg.

This is a wonderful base to which you can add adaptogens (herbal supplements to relieve stress), but please consult an Ayurvedic practitioner prior to doing this, as these herbs should be used as part of a protocol rather than sporadically.

THE APOTHECARY

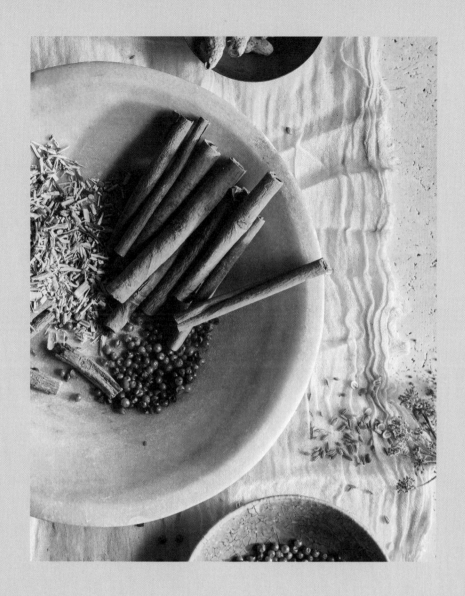

Ayurvedic first-aid kit

By accessing 'nature's medicine cabinet', also known as your spice rack, you have the ability to heal many common health ailments without the need for pharmaceutical products. As a species, we survived for thousands of years on plant medicine alone. Now you have the power to access this wisdom to become your own healer.

Anxiety:

o   Make a tea of ½ teaspoon valerian root (known as tagar) in 1 cup (250 ml/8½ fl oz) hot water.

o   Make a tea of ½ teaspoon brahmi and ½ teaspoon tulsi in 1 cup (250 ml/8½ fl oz) hot water.

o   Drink 1 cup (250 ml/8½ fl oz) orange juice with 1 teaspoon honey and a pinch of nutmeg.

o   Use meditation and pranayama to slow the breath and come back to the body.

Asthma/wheezing/coughing fit:

o   Boil 1 cup licorice tea and continuously sip until coughing ceases.

Bites/stings:

o   Apply a paste of bruised coriander (cilantro) or neem leaves to the affected area.

o   Dilute ¼ teaspoon neem oil in 1 teaspoon coconut oil and apply.

Bleeding (topical):

o   Cover the open wound in ground turmeric powder to coagulate the blood and stop the bleeding. The antibiotic properties of turmeric also help to disinfect the wound and promote healing.

Bleeding (internal):

o   Drink 1 cup (250 ml/8½ fl oz) of either pomegranate or cranberry juice. Both of these fruits are astringent by nature, meaning they can restrict the flow of blood.

Burns and sunburn:

o   Immediately apply cold waater or ice to the affected area.

o   Cover with aloe vera gel or coconut oil.

o   Bruised coriander (cilantro) pulp is also useful.

Colds:

o   Use turmeric and garlic in cooking, as these are powerful antibiotics.

o   Mix 1 teaspoon honey with ⅛ teaspoon turmeric and take between meals.

o   Brew 2.5 cm (1 in) piece of grated ginger root in 5 cups (1.25 litres/42 fl oz) water and sip throughout the day, or drink the respiratory tea (see page 181).

Constipation:

o   Mix ½ teaspoon psyllium husk in 1 cup of water. Drink on an empty stomach.

o   Take ¼ teaspoon triphala on the tongue, sip a cup of water to swallow.

Dehydration:

o Add a pinch of salt and a pinch of jaggery or coconut sugar to 1 cup of water. Drink up to 3 cups throughout the day to increase your intake of electrolytes.

Earache:

o Dilute 5 drops of neem oil and 5 drops of tea-tree oil in 20 drops of sesame oil; keep in a small glass jar and apply morning and night with a cotton swab.

Fever:

o Chew 1 teaspoon fennel seeds.

o Make a tea with 5–10 mint leaves in 1 cup (250 ml/8½ fl oz) warm water.

o Apply a paste of bruised coriander (cilantro) leaves or a cool facecloth to the forehead.

o Avoid eating.

Hangover:

o Drink 1 cup (250 ml/8½ fl oz) orange juice with 1 teaspoon lime juice and a pinch of ground cumin.

Hiccups:

o Mix 1 teaspoon honey and 1 teaspoon castor oil, then dip the tip of a teaspoon into the mix and lick it every few minutes.

Headache:

o Massage peppermint oil into the temples.

o Make a tea of ½ teaspoon valerian root (known as tagar) in 1 cup (250 ml/8½ fl oz) hot water.

o Drink CCF tea (see page 130).

o Chew ½ teaspoon ajwain seeds for up to 3 minutes, then swallow.

Inflammation:

o Drink dandelion tea, which is a natural diuretic and will help to reduce the swelling and flush the excess liquid out.

Insomnia:

o For a blissful night's sleep, make one of the suggested moon milks (see page 184).

o Make a paste of ½ teaspoon ghee and ½ teaspoon nutmeg powder, and massage into the temples.

Irritated eyes:

o External use: boil 1 teaspoon coriander (cilantro) seeds in 1 cup (250 ml/8½ fl oz) water for 15 minutes, cool, then apply over closed eyes.

o Internal use: boil 1 teaspoon Triphala in 1 cup (250 ml/8½ fl oz) water for 3–5 minutes, allow the tea to cool, then strain it through a paper coffee filter, paper towel or cheesecloth to remove all of the powder grains – rinse the eyes as needed.

Nausea (morning sickness, motion sickness, food poisoning):

o Brew 2.5 cm (1 in) piece of ginger root, grated, in 5 cups (1.25 litres/42 fl oz) water and sip throughout the day.

o Eat freshly grated ginger with a squeeze of lime.

o Fill a small vegetable capsule (available at some chemists and organic or health food stores) with ground ginger powder and take with water before travelling or flying.

Nosebleed:

o Inhale a few drops of pomegranate or cranberry juice using an eyedropper.

Pain (period pain, joint pain, headache):

o Chew ½ teaspoon ajwain seeds every few hours, or as needed. Chew for 3–5 minutes, then swallow.

Reflux/indigestion:

o Chew ½ teaspoon fennel seeds or cumin seeds.

o Drink CCF tea (see page 130).

Sinus congestion:

o Chew a piece of pippali (long black pepper) or a few whole peppercorns to relieve congestion.

o Melt 1 teaspoon ghee, wash your hands and use the pinky finger to massage the ghee into the inner cavities of the nostril to moisturise and relieve dryness.

o Do facial steaming with 2 drops of eucalyptus oil (see page 97).

Sweating (excessive):

o Infuse a pot of hot water with 1 tablespoon sage leaves, leave overnight and sip throughout the day. Sage contains astringent properties that constrict the sweat glands and reduce perspiration. Sage is also an antibacterial and antifungal that restricts the growth of bacteria.

Tooth decay:

o Chew 1 teaspoon white sesame seeds for 5 minutes each morning, then brush your teeth with the pulp of the seeds. The calcium content will help to restore the tooth enamel and impart whiter, brighter teeth.

Golden nectar

The union of honey, turmeric and black pepper create a healing force willing and able to combat a plethora of health issues such as respiratory disorders, digestive issues, infections, allergies, inflammation, all types of pain, skin and liver conditions, amongst others. This is nature's finest medicine, packed full of anti-inflammatory, antioxidant, antifungal, and antibacterial properties.

Makes 1 cup

1 cup of raw, organic honey

1 tablespoon ground turmeric

¼ teaspoon black pepper

Mix all ingredients in a glass jar, store out of direct sunlight.

It can be taken orally by taking 1/2 teaspoon on the tongue as needed, or used topically.

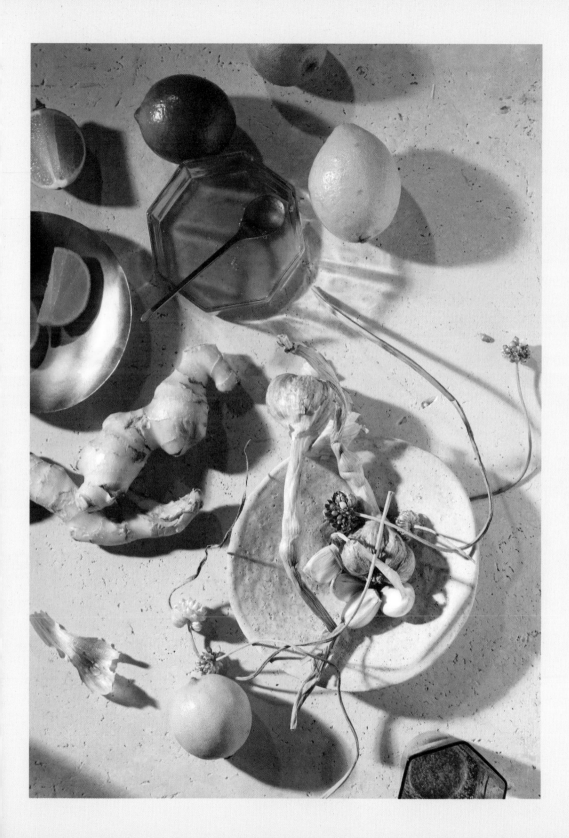

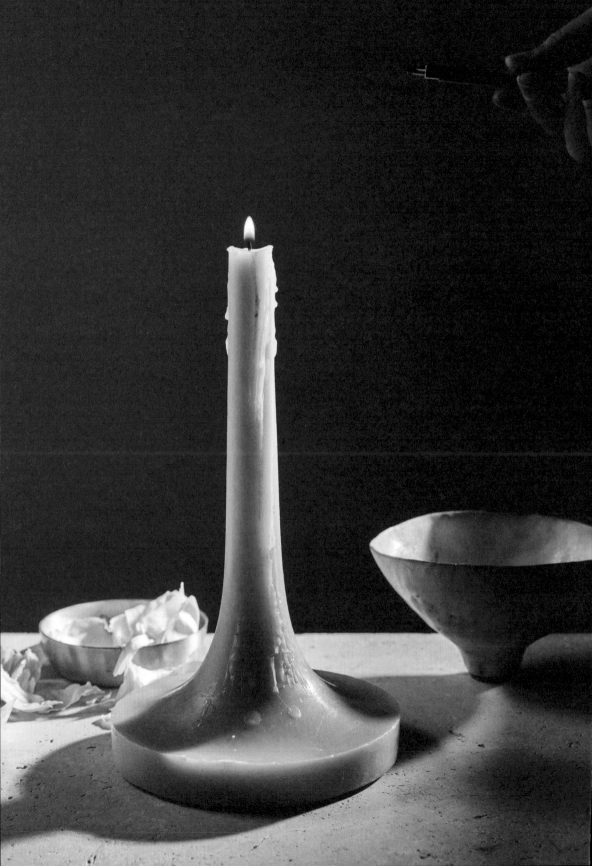

Glossary

Abhyanga	A full body massage using warm herbal oil to balance all of the Doshas, improve circulation and detoxification, heal and prevent disease, and centre the mind.
Agni	Known as 'the digestive fire', which is responsible for digestion, absorption and assimilation of all that is consumed (including food, nutrients and everything perceived via the sensory portals – eyes, ears, nose, tongue and skin). Agni's function is to transform matter into tissues, energy and consciousness.
Ahimsa	The philosophy of non-violence towards all living, sentient beings.
Alkaline	A pH measure of over 7 that creates a protective environment within the body where disease cannot exist.
Ama	A toxic residue that can accumulate in the body when food, herbs, emotions or experiences are not fully processed, digested or assimilated. Ama often resides within the weakest or compromised parts of the body; this is where disease is bred.
Ayurveda	An ancient system of healing translated as 'the science of life' that dates back 5000 years and is known as the original system of healthcare, with deep roots in Indian Vedic culture.
Dinacharya	Translated as 'daily routine', designed to provide structure and to align our bodies with the natural rhythms of nature while nourishing the body, mind and spirit through self-care, bathing, meditation, yoga, spirituality, regular meals and sleep practices.
Dosha	A body of functional energy known as either Vata, Pitta and Kapha, comprising certain elements (Space, Air, Fire, Water, Earth) found in nature and within the body, which is used to identify imbalances and restore harmony.
Holistic	A system designed to consider all facets of disease manifestation and treatment protocols, including diet, lifestyle, social, mental and physical factors, where the root cause is investigated and removed, rather than treating symptoms alone.
Homeostasis	A state in which the body is balanced; the base level before disease or stress occurs.
Kapha	One of the three Doshas (functional energies); Kapha is comprised of the Earth and Water elements and governs structure and stability; it is heavy, slow, cool, oily, smooth, dense, soft, stable, gross and cloudy.

Malas	The three forms of waste produced by the body in order to effectively eliminate and detoxify, including urine, faeces and sweat.
Ojas	A tangible liquid or life-force energy surrounding every cell that offers protection and resistance, creating the basis of physical strength, stamina, longevity and immunity. Ojas is the end product of healthy digestion.
Pakti	The process of cooking food to aid digestion.
Pancha Maha Boutas	Known as the 'Five Great Elements', which include Space, Air, Fire, Water and Earth, of which everything on earth is made up in varying quantities.
Pitta	One of the three Doshas (functional energies); Pitta is comprised of the Fire and Water elements, and governs transformation; it is hot, sharp, oily and spreading.
Prabhava	An innate intelligence that inspires a change within the body that cannot be explained by logic or reason.
Prakriti	The unique Doshic constitution (Vata, Pitta, Kapha) of an individual determined at conception, which inspires their physical, emotional and mental disposition.
Prana	Vital life-force energy ingested through breath, as well as pure foods and clean water, that fuels the body and mind to inspire longevity, clarity of mind, intelligence, perception and fluid communication.
Pranayama	Yogic breathing practices that carry Prana throughout the body and mind to increase awareness, consciousness and mental clarity while releasing stagnant energy from within to prepare for meditation.
Rasa	Translated as 'taste' or 'flavour', relating both to food and life itself; the juiciness of an experience that promotes internal joy, which feeds the body and spirit.
Rasayana	A substance or experience that nourishes Rasa and in turn strengthens all of the bodily tissues, the immune system and the mind.
Ritucharya	Translated as 'seasonal routine', designed to promote balance throughout the changing cycles of the year based on our environment and the ever-changing patterns of nature and the seasons.
Sadhana	Anything that is practised with awareness, discipline and the intention of spiritual growth.
Sanskrit	Classical language of India in which Vedic texts were recorded. Known as 'the perfect language', every letter and word is designed to resonate a potent vibration.

Sneha	Translated with two direct meanings, 'oil' and 'love', referring to the application of oil, or abhyanga, as a practice of love.
Srotas	A physical or energetic pathway or channel that carries substances or energy from one place to another within the body.
Symbiotic	To live harmoniously with multiple species or as part of nature without any disruption to the fundamental aspects of the environment.
Svastha	Described as a state of optimum health and wellbeing gained through having balanced Doshas, a calm mind, healthy bodily tissues, effective elimination processes and strong Agni.
Tapas	The power associated with the confidence to shake off any dispelling beliefs about yourself, your potential or the reasoning behind your action. In Sanskrit, Tapas means 'to heat or burn up', referring to the way discipline burns off the space for negative self-talk and self-imposed limitations.
Tamasic	One of the three universal energies (Sattva, Tamas, Rajas) that relates to heavy, dormant or destructive energy.
Trataka	A form of meditation that involves open-eye gazing at a small flame.
Tridoshic	Pacifying or balancing for all three Doshas: Vata, Pitta and Kapha.
Vata	One of the three Doshas (functional energies); Vata is comprised of the Space and Air elements and governs movement and communication; it is light, cold, dry, rough, mobile, subtle and clear.
Vedic	A period of time in India (approximately 1750–500 BC) in which the Vedas (original texts on Ayurveda and yoga) were composed.
Vikriti	The current doshic constitution (Vata, Pitta, Kapha) of an individual, determined by any imbalances within the body and mind.
Yoga	Translated as 'union', relating to the physical practice of asanas (postures) designed to unite the body and mind to strengthen meditation while also promoting the flexibility and strength of the physical body.

Index

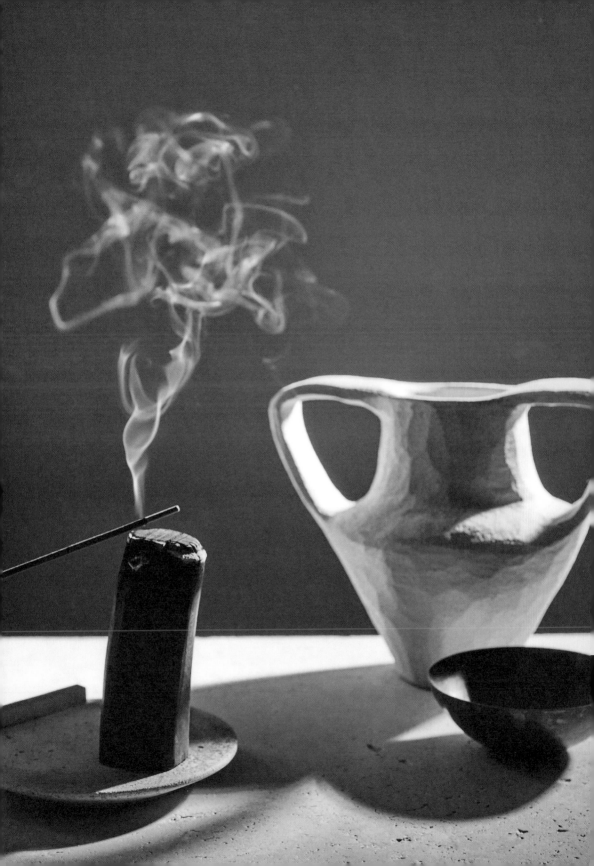

About the author

After a life-long exploration of alternative living, sustainability, natural medicine, plant-based cooking, yoga & meditation, Chasca Summerville embarked on the journey of Ayurveda while exploring the diverse and colourful lands of India in 2017 on a mission to deepen her practice of yoga. Instantly connecting with the ancient science of Ayurveda, she put her career as a filmmaker on hold to study, and obtained a Diploma of Ayurvedic Lifestyle Consultation from the Ayurveda College in Byron Bay, Australia.

With a passion for natural healing of the body and mind, Chasca's mission is to share the knowledge of Ayurveda to inspire others to understand themselves deeply, to establish a lifestyle that serves our best opportunity for true health, to release emotional limitations, while understanding the interconnectedness of the mind and body paradigm, and to find our place within nature so that we can live harmoniously with the land and minimise our carbon footprint.

In an age where life is lived in the fast lane, Chasca believes that Ayurveda has never been more necessary and that in order to nourish ourselves we need the wisdom of Ayurveda to guide us towards a wholesome diet, a complimentary lifestyle, self-care practices that nourish the deepest layers of our being, establish a centre of balance, and keep us grounded when everything around us seems never to slow down.

Abundant with passion, creativity, romance and liberation, Chasca's experience of Ayurveda has inspired her to share her perspective through these same forms of creativity, bringing a modern voice to an ancient science with the hope that this may resonate, and speak to society in a way that will inspire people to return to ancient ways of living that align with the natural world in order to serve ourselves and our planet.

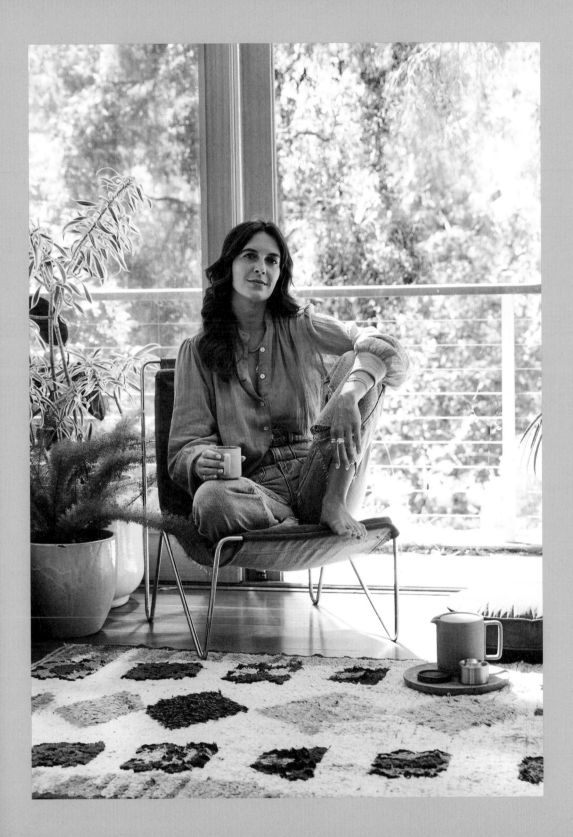

With gratitude

I would like to heartfully acknowledge the Australian Aboriginal and Torres Strait Islander peoples as the traditional custodians of the land from which I have been blessed to write this book, amongst the majesty of the eucalyptus and wattle trees; and to all indigenous peoples all over this vast world - the naturalists, the wild healers and those who are able to find joy through living in harmony with mother nature. It is through your teachings that we are able to find our place within our ecosystem and live a life as nature intended. My deepest respect is with you.

Those who have dutifully passed on the sacred wisdom of Ayurveda, including the teachers, healers, gurus, sages, rishis and to everyone who has taken a chance at exploring this way of living, including you, the readers of this book - thank you. I feel amongst many, infinitely blessed to have stumbled across this seemingly perfect way of living.

I wouldn't have had the knowledge or expertise to write this book without the guidance of my mentor, Professor Jason Chandler, who has dedicated his life to passing on the vast and complex nuances of Ayurveda. To everyone at the Ayurveda College in Byron Bay, thank you for your tireless work and dedication to supporting everyone who comes through your doors.

The wonderful team at Hardie Grant, including my publisher Alice, who shares my passion for the Art of Living, I am eternally grateful for your support and the opportunity to bring this book to life. And to the colourful team of creatives who turned my words into magic along with the wonderful brands that contributed to our photoshoot, including All That Remains is Love, Hara the Label, Rollas, SolidTeknics, Maison Balzac, Cisco & the Sun, and Cultivar.

To my beloved community that surrounds, inspires and motivates me to push through and surpass limitations, especially to my best friends Victoria Bolton & Sophia Robinson who have been there to support and encourage me from day one. Lastly to my beautiful family, who have always been my greatest teachers and inspiration and created a stable base from which to catch me when I fall, and to my mother for inspiring me to believe I could be anyone I wanted to be. I love you all.

There is no greater force to inspire us than through overcoming hardship or illness in one's own story. In saying that, I am grateful for all of the challenges I have faced and learned from. My motivating force in writing this book is to inspire you to understand and connect with yourself deeply, so that you can find the bounty in your hardships and experience liberation through this.

MEDICAL DISCLAIMER

The practices described in this book do not take into account the reader's individual health, medical, physical, psychological, or emotional situation or needs and therefore may not be safe for all people.

The information provided in this book is designed to provide helpful information on the subjects discussed. The author and publisher are not medical professionals and cannot give medical advice or diagnosis. This book is not meant to be used, nor should it be used, to diagnose or treat any medical condition. The reader should, before acting or using any of this information, consider the appropriateness of this information having regard to their own personal situation and needs. For diagnosis or treatment of any medical problem, the reader must consult a medical professional. The author and publisher expressly disclaim all and any liability to any person in respect of anything and of the consequences of anything done or omitted to be done by any person in reliance, whether in whole or part, upon the whole or any part of the contents of this book and/or any website(s) referred to in it. Nothing in this medical disclaimer will limit any liabilities of the author or publisher in any way that is prohibited by law, or exclude any liabilities that may not be excluded by law. If anything in this disclaimer is unenforceable, illegal, or void, it is severed and the rest of the disclaimer remains in force. References are provided for informational purposes only and do not constitute endorsement of any websites or other sources.

Published in 2021 by Hardie Grant Books,
an imprint of Hardie Grant Publishing

Hardie Grant Books (Melbourne)
Building 1, 658 Church Street
Richmond, Victoria 3121

Hardie Grant Books (London)
5th & 6th Floors
52–54 Southwark Street
London SE1 1UN

hardiegrantbooks.com

 A catalogue record for this
book is available from the
National Library of Australia

Ayurvedic Rituals
ISBN 978 1 74379 706 8

10 9 8 7 6 5 4 3 2 1

Commissioning Editor: Alice Hardie-Grant
Editor: Marg Bowman
Design Manager: Mietta Yans
Designer: Ashley Simonetto
Photographer: Armelle Habib
Stylist: Stephanie Stamatis
Production Manager: Todd Rechner
Colour reproduction by Splitting Image Colour Studio
Printed in China by Leo Paper Products LTD.

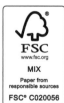 The paper this book is printed on is from FSC® - certified forests and other
sources. FSC® promotes environmentally responsible, socially beneficial and
economically viable management of the world's forests.

*Hardie Grant acknowledges the Traditional Owners of the country on which we work,
the Wurundjeri people of the Kulin nation and the Gadigal people of the Eora nation,
and recognises their continuing connection to the land, waters and culture.
We pay our respects to their Elders past, present and emerging.*